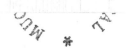
Clinical judgement and decision-making

in Nursing and interprofessional healthcare

In loving memory of Lau Wai Cheng, my father, whose energy, vision, self sacrifice, sense of duty and practical wisdom ensured that my nine brothers and sisters and I all benefited from and valued education as a means of developing character and transforming our lives.

Clinical judgement and decision-making

in Nursing and interprofessional healthcare

Edited by

Mooi Standing

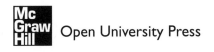 Open University Press

Open University Press
McGraw-Hill Education
McGraw-Hill House
Shoppenhangers Road
Maidenhead
Berkshire
England
SL6 2QL

email: enquiries@openup.co.uk
world wide web: www.openup.co.uk

and
Two Penn Plaza, New York, NY 10121-2289, USA

First published 2010

A catalogue record of this book is available from the British Library

ISBN13: 978-0-33-523626-8 (pb) 978-0-33-523625-1 (hb)
ISBN10: 0-33-523626-X (pb) 0-33-523625-1 (hb)

Library of Congress Cataloging-in-Publication Data
CIP data has been applied for

Typeset by Aptara Inc., India
Printed in the UK by Bell and Bain, Glasgow

Fictitous names of companies, products, people, characters and/or data that
may be used herein (in case studies or in examples) are not intended to
represent any real individual, company, product or event.

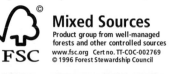

Mixed Sources
Product group from well-managed
forests and other controlled sources
www.fsc.org   Cert no. TT-COC-002769
© 1996 Forest Stewardship Council

The **McGraw·Hill** Companies

Contents

List of figures

List of tables

About the editor

Mooi Standing, BSc, MA, PhD, RGN, RMN, CPN, RNT is a Principal Lecturer and Quality head in nursing and applied clinical studies at Canterbury Christ Church University. Mooi practised mental health and general nursing in various hospital and community settings before becoming a lecturer, and has been involved in nurse education for over 20 years. Mooi is actively involved in the development of overseas collaborative nursing programmes at undergraduate and post-qualifying levels. She is the designated Programme Director and Academic Link Manager for the collaborative BSc (Hons) Nursing Studies, Malaysia.

In addition, she teaches and supervises nursing students from undergraduate to PhD level studies including designing and facilitating experiental judgement and decision-making workshops on the MSc Interprofessional Health and Social Care. Mooi has established her professional and academic standing through her PhD research on the perception by nursing students and the development of clinical decision-making skills of nursing students. She has since developed and published a new critical framework for applying hermeneutic phenomenology, nine modes of practice on a cognitive continuum of decision-making, and a matrix model on the perception of nursing and decision-making skills.

Mooi is also an accredited Nursing and Midwifery Council (NMC) reviewer who applies her expertise and experience in approving, monitoring, and assuring the quality of nursing programmes throughout the United Kingdom. Mooi also provides external consultancy in curriculum development assessment and quality enhancement both nationally and internationally.

Contributors

Kate Dewar RGN, RNT, MSc (Nursing) is an independent higher education lecturer, teaching in both interprofessional and unidisciplinary Masters level programmes. She has particular interest in all issues associated with advanced practice including the critical thinking skills that underpin it. When previously working as a Senior Lecturer at Canterbury Christ Church University, she developed programmes and courses which supported advanced level nursing practice, and undertook various research projects related to these developments. Kate's current doctoral research concerns the theory and knowledge associated with advanced level practice.

Elizabeth Duck is an Advanced Practitioner/Therapy Radiographer and Clinical Lead for breast cancer patients attending the radiotherapy department. She is responsible for imaging and treatment field planning. Elizabeth has taken part in the Society of Radiographers' pilot study for accreditation of advanced practitioners. She is currently undertaking research on oncologists' decision-making processes within the field of breast radiotherapy as part of a higher degree dissertation.

Peter Ellis is a Senior Lecturer at Canterbury Christ Church University. His main teaching interests are evidence-based practice and research methods, epidemiology and public health medicine, nephrology nursing, ethics and care management. He is widely published in renal nursing and epidemiology of renal disease, healthcare ethics and health service management. He also teaches, monitors, and examines on Managing Care for the Open University. Peter was Senior Nurse Renal Outpatients and Research Projects Manager in the Renal Unit at King's College Hospital, London, and is a visiting lecturer at various universities in London.

Roger Goldsmith is a Senior Lecturer at Canterbury Christ Church University. His clinical expertise lies in Accident and Emergency Nursing which he continues to practise. Roger teaches on the pre-registration interprofessional learning programme, focusing on clinical science and care of acute and critically ill patients. He also teaches advanced practice in minor injury and minor illness management.

Hesham Hassan is a Consultant Psychiatrist with a vast experience of psychiatry in various health settings. He is employed by the Kent and Medway Partnership Trust. He practises in a town and rural community mental health team developing and applying new frames of working to care for adults with severe and enduring mental illness.

Carolyn Jackson is Head of Department for Nursing and Applied Clinical Studies at Canterbury Christ Church University. With a career spanning almost three decades in nursing in the UK, the Mediterranean and Australasia, Carolyn's main concerns are to advance nursing practice through education, scholarship and practice development initiatives. Her main interests are in management and leadership, education, advanced practice, health policy and interprofessional practice.

Douglas MacInnes, Reader in Mental Health, is a mental health nurse whose main expertise concerns working with mentally disordered offenders. He undertook a PhD at Guy's Kings and St Thomas' School of Medicine, King's College, University of London. The dissertation examined the views and experiences of the caregivers of people with schizophrenia. Subsequently, he also completed an MSc in Cognitive Behaviour Therapy. Douglas is involved in the teaching of research skills (from diploma to PhD students) as well as undertaking and supervising research projects. He is also seconded by the local health trust to work in clinical practice as a cognitive therapist for one day a week. Douglas's recent research has centred on the themes of cognitive therapy, family work, illness beliefs, working with mentally disordered offenders, and examining the stigma faced by those with mental health problems. His research has been supported and funded locally by Health and Social Care Trusts and Nationally by the Department of Health.

Susan Plummer is a Principal Lecturer in mental health at Canterbury Christ Church University. Susan was awarded a Medical Research Council Special Training Fellowship in the Health of the Public and Health Services Research in 2001. She has participated in many research projects in mental health at the Institute of Psychiatry, London and co-authored a number of related journal articles/book chapters. She has presented at conferences in the United States, Australia and Europe. She continues practice in primary mental health nursing two days a month.

Antonio Sama is a Senior Lecturer at Canterbury Christ Church University. He currently lectures on the MSc Interprofessional Health and Social Care including: judgement and decision-making; psychodynamics of interprofessional practice/organizational dynamics; and advanced collaborative practice models. Antonio's interests include: organizational changes in social care; evaluating innovations in social policy and social services; comparative research and education in European social work; and the history of professional organizational consultancy.

Michael Standing obtained a PGCEA, Six Category Intervention Analysis Trainers Certificate, and an MSc in Social Research (quantitative and qualitative methods) at the University of Surrey (Education, Human Potential

Research Project, and Sociology departments). He combined and applied these influences to lead the development and facilitation of an innovative community mental health nursing programme for a consortium of six Kent health authorities. He also led an applied psychosocial sciences team at City University (School of Nursing and Midwifery) in integrating social sciences, research methods, interpersonal, management, leadership and learning/ teaching skills throughout the curriculum. More recently Michael has been adapting to a disability but continues to offer others support and mentoring, from home, in their scholarly endeavours.

Introduction

The main audience for this book will be the nursing profession including advanced practitioners, registered nurses engaging in professional development, clinical nurse managers, specialist nurses, midwives, community nurses, and nurse educators. Its focus on the theory and practice of clinical judgement and decision-making will also interest other healthcare professionals given the interprofessional nature of many decisions. Most authors are experienced nurses but there are contributions by a radiographer (Chapter 7) and a psychiatrist (Chapter 9), and whole systems theory (Chapter 3) emphasizes collaborative, integrated healthcare. Chapter 10 applies decision theory to evaluate a general practitioner's diagnostic skills, and then offers a new interprofessional healthcare model. There is, therefore, an interprofessional thread throughout the book, and much of the theory presented is applicable to a wide range of health professionals.

The book is intended as essential reading to support higher education nursing/interprofessional continuing professional development programmes, including postgraduate decision-making, research, evidence-based, and reflective practice modules. It will also appeal to practitioners with inquiring minds and a commitment to their professional development, who wish to supplement informal work-based learning with new ways of exploring, understanding and applying clinical judgement and decision-making skills. It aims to engage the interest of any reader who is prepared to question and reflect on clinical practice with a view to developing their understanding and expertise, which can enhance the quality of patient-centred care. Elements of the book may also be suitable as recommended reading for students on pre-registration programmes, for example, Chapter 1 refers to a study of nursing students' development in decision-making.

Nursing is a practice-orientated profession in using clinical skills to promote health, supplement individuals', families' and local communities' self-caring abilities, and relieve pain and suffering where necessary throughout the human lifecycle. Sound clinical judgement and decision-making skills are vital to perform this complex role effectively in a wide range of challenging healthcare contexts. They require the ongoing development and synthesis of relevant theoretical and research knowledge, self-awareness, interpersonal, and practical skills (Higgs and Titchen 2001). The structure and organization of the book are intended to enhance the reader's personal understanding, application and integration of theoretical and practical considerations in this respect.

The first five chapters present relevant, contemporary theory, and recent research findings in clinical judgement and decision-making. The second half of the book presents advanced nurse practitioners' accounts, reflections and analysis (e.g. mapping interventions against decision theory) of their clinical judgements and decision-making in a variety of hospital and community healthcare settings. A patient's account of care received for a serious illness is also included to provide a patient-centred perspective, and reflecting on this experience culminates in the creation of a new 'reflexive-pragmatism' model of interprofessional healthcare. It also illustrates that clinical practice is not simply a place to apply the findings of existing theory and research; it is also a place where new insights and experiences can be described which help to generate new models of understanding. In this way, theory and practice are mutually energizing influences in the book.

Chapter 1 presents the findings of a longitudinal phenomenological study from which a matrix model is derived combining nurses' personal, theoretical conceptions of nursing with their practical experience and perceptions of developing clinical decision-making skills. The findings support a synthesis of reflective and evidence-based practice within ethical and professional patient-centred care. Chapter 2 includes an extensive literature review of the intellectual and personality attributes of advanced practitioners needed for a wide range of clinical competences and role functions. Chapter 3 looks beyond practitioners' perceptions to the organizational contexts in which they work and advocates the understanding and application of whole systems theory using creative thinking skills and interprofessional collaboration for effective care delivery. Chapter 4 explores the importance of lifelong learning in clinical judgement and decision-making skills and ways of enhancing informal work-based learning opportunities. A case is also made for creating a participative interprofessional community of learning in formal continuing professional development programmes to integrate theory and practice. Chapter 5 explores the development of cognitive continuum theory in combining intuitive/experiential and analytic/rational decision approaches. A new revised cognitive continuum is developed for nurses and other health professionals, relating nine modes of practice to patient-centred tasks, and correspondence (practical) and coherence (logical) competence are applied to evaluate judgement and decision-making. Each of the above theoretical and research perspectives encourages in-depth understanding of applying critical thinking skills, in patient-centred judgement and decision-making in healthcare contexts.

Chapters 6 to 10 present real case study situations that are analysed using the theory and research referred to in Chapters 1 to 5. Chapter 6 focuses on prioritizing skills for a patient in a nurse-led minor injury unit who has fallen and fractured a bone in her hand. Chapter 7 focuses on interprofessional accountability when a radiotherapist discovers a procedure requested by an oncologist is not supported by the patient's pathology. Chapter 8 explores short- and long-term risk assessment and management strategies within forensic mental health care. Chapter 9 presents a reflection of clinical supervision regarding the supervisee's judgements, decisions and interventions in assessing a patient with suicidal intentions. Chapter 10 describes experiences of receiving urgent medical care over a ten-year period, and the concepts of correspondence and coherence competence (from cognitive continuum theory) are applied to evaluate decision-making. In reflecting on ways to enhance the development and application of decision-making skills, a new reflexive-pragmatism model is created for interprofessional healthcare. The discussion of the case studies will highlight decision-making themes that are relevant to other areas of healthcare, and readers will be encouraged to relate the contents to their own particular area of clinical practice.

The most important emphasis of the book is to challenge and enable readers to reflect on and enhance their clinical practice by presenting theory and research which they can understand and relate to, and to present extensive examples of how to integrate the theory and practice of clinical judgement and decision-making via practitioners' review of real clinical scenarios. Currently, there is no other book so strongly practice-orientated with extensive input from a wide range of advanced practitioners, sharing their experiences, helping bridge a theory–practice gap, and providing unique insights into their clinical judgement and decision-making processes. Reflective activities are included throughout the book to encourage active participation in the learning process and test out the feasibility of the ideas presented. The book also contains models, diagrams and self-assessment tools which readers can apply to enhance clinical practice, and provides useful reference sources for formal studies and their continuing professional development.

Reference

Higgs, J. and Titchen, A. (2001) *Practice Knowledge and Expertise*. Oxford: Butterworth Heinemann.

1 Perceptions of clinical decision-making: a matrix model

Mooi Standing

Overview

This chapter defines and discusses clinical decision-making in relation to cultural influences, professional identity, decision theory and a matrix model that cross-references nurses' perceptions of clinical decision-making with their conceptual understanding of nursing. Although most of the discussion and examples relate to nursing, the issues are relevant to other health professionals. The requirement for all health professionals to be publicly accountable in demonstrating sound clinical judgement and decision-making sets the context against which these skills, together with critical thinking and problem solving, are discussed. Normative, prescriptive and descriptive decision-making models are related to contrasting scientific and experiential processes (and sources of evidence) to support clinical decisions. Benner's 'novice to expert' model of clinical expertise is critiqued and a matrix model, derived from a longitudinal phenomenological study of nurses' developmental journey, acquiring and applying clinical decision-making skills, is presented. Reflective activities invite readers to relate the matrix model to their experience and perceptions of clinical decision-making. The matrix model is then critiqued with reference to decision theory.

Objectives

- Appreciate how clinical decision-making defines the nature of healthcare professions
- Describe problem solving, critical thinking, clinical judgement, and clinical decision-making
- Distinguish between normative, prescriptive and descriptive decision-making models
- Compare and contrast a 'novice to expert' model of skill acquisition with the matrix model
- Identify different types and sources of evidence, and ways of processing clinical decisions
- Consider common errors in clinical judgement/decision-making and how to prevent them

• Reflect on development needs regarding clinical judgement and decision-making skills

Background

The importance of developing and using effective clinical decision-making skills was reinforced by a National Health Service (NHS) reform that introduced a system of clinical governance to facilitate quality-assured healthcare and greater public accountability of health professionals (DH 1998). This was supported by calls for evidence-based decisions to raise standards of care, accompanied by performance-related pay to encourage health professionals to review and adapt their practice in line with organizational and managerial changes (NHS Executive 1999; DH 1999). The NHS Plan identified targets to increase public access to high quality healthcare, established criteria to monitor achievement of targets via NHS Service Frameworks, and advocated a flexible multidisciplinary workforce to improve the coordination, efficiency, and effectiveness of health services (DH 2000). The concept of 'working together, learning together' through lifelong learning acknowledged the ongoing education and training implications of developing health professionals' core skills in communication, information processing, teamwork, and clinical competence. Partnerships between Workforce Development Confederations and higher education institutions were established to tailor education to health service providers' requirements in matching skills to local clinical demands (DH 2001).

Background summary

• In the United Kingdom a policy of healthcare for all, freely available at the point of delivery, is achieved via the NHS, the largest employer in the country, publicly funded by taxation.
• Government-led NHS reform aims to improve its efficiency, quality, and cost effectiveness on behalf of the public who elected them and whose taxes indirectly pay for services.
• Organizational changes such as setting health targets and clinical governance mean that the actions of health professionals are subject to greater managerial and public scrutiny.
• Health professions continue to self-regulate standards of practice but, as NHS employees, practitioners are also assessed through quality audit and individual performance appraisal.
• The increased public accountability of health professionals means that clinical judgements, decisions and interventions must be explained, justified, and defended when challenged.
• Changes in health professionals' education complement NHS reform by linking theory to evidence-based practice, developing skills, and encouraging interprofessional learning.

The above factors have implications for reviewing the role and function of health professionals (Chapter 2), adapting the organization and management of NHS services (Chapter 3), and, continuing interprofessional development in clinical judgement and decision-making (Chapter 4).

The impact of cultural change and NHS reform also poses a challenge to the professional identity and autonomy of healthcare workers in accommodating government health targets, principles of evidence-based practice, and public accountability for their clinical judgements and decisions. This chapter explores these issues in relation to nursing, the largest professional group in the NHS, but the points raised are also relevant to other health professionals.

Nursing, clinical decision-making and professional identity

For many years the following definition was thought to convey the essential nature and professional identity of nursing:

> The unique function of the nurse is to assist the individual, sick or well, in the performance of those activities contributing to health, or its recovery (or to a peaceful death) that he would perform unaided if he had the necessary strength, will or knowledge.
>
> (Henderson 1966: 15)

Thirty-three years later the (then) regulating body for nursing stated that this 'definition of nursing has not been bettered' (UKCC 1999: 15). Indeed, Henderson's patient-centred, needs-focused, collaborative, and goal-directed emphasis appears as relevant now as it was then but the cognitive skills necessary to determine and demonstrate how best to 'assist the individual' were not made explicit. More recently the Royal College of Nursing has redefined nursing as:

> The use of clinical judgement in the provision of care to enable people to improve, maintain, or recover health to cope with health problems, and to achieve the best possible quality of life whatever their disease or disability, until death.
>
> (RCN 2003: 3)

Both definitions support the view that nursing, 'as a human science focuses on life and health as humanly experienced' (Pilkington 2005: 98). However, the emphasis upon 'use of clinical judgement' distinguishes the RCN definition from earlier versions and shows how nursing is continually adapting to cultural change, including NHS reform, in order to meet new challenges and role requirements that enhance the quality of care and accountability for clinical decision-making.

The subtle shift in focus from what nurses do, to how they think about what they need to do, places clinical judgement and decision-making skills at the forefront of nurses' professional identity. This is also true for other professions since comparing judgements and decisions made by different healthcare professionals enables the identification of their distinctive contribution to patient care. The implications for nurse education led to reform of pre-registration programmes through the introduction of practice-orientated curricula designed to equip nurses with relevant clinical skills so they are 'fit for practice and purpose' (UKCC 2001). In other words theoretical knowledge is of limited value unless it helps to inform and guide high standards of patient care that is responsive and adjusted to individual needs and circumstances. This capacity to integrate theory and practice underpins the notion of the nurse as a 'knowledgeable-doer' (Benner 1984) and it is also needed 'to justify, explain and defend judgements and decisions' (Dowding and Thompson 2002: 190).

Hence, the Nursing and Midwifery Council (the current regulating body) require pre-registration nursing programmes to prepare nurses who can 'demonstrate sound clinical decision-making' (NMC 2004: 33) and these skills are internationally acknowledged as core competences in nurse education (Gonzalez and Wagenaar 2005). All registered nurses and midwives in the United Kingdom are bound by a code of conduct which states 'As a professional, you are personally accountable for actions and omissions in your practice and must always be able to justify your decisions' and, 'You must deliver care based on the best available evidence or best practice' (NMC 2008: 1). Other health professions' regulatory bodies stipulate similar requirements for their practitioners. Clarifying what is meant by the terms clinical judgement and decision-making is, therefore, needed in healthcare.

Problem solving, critical thinking, clinical judgement, and clinical decision-making

Healthcare involves addressing health problems and the nursing process is a well-established problem solving approach to systematically assess, diagnose, plan, implement and evaluate individualized care using intellectual, interpersonal and technical skills (Yura and Walsh 1973). Each stage of the nursing process requires the use of judgement and decision-making and this is more effective when critical thinking skills are applied. Indeed, criticisms of the nursing process focus mainly on its uncritical application: Parse (1981) argued it was too mechanistic; Hurst et al. (1991) reported that the more cognitively demanding planning and evaluation stages were neglected; Corcoran-Perry and Narayan (1995: 70) asserted that it 'delineated neither the underlying thinking processes nor the specific knowledge involved'; and Benner et al. (1996) claimed it led to the routine use of standardized care plans that militated against individualized care planning. The development of clinical judgement and decision-making skills can, therefore, complement the nursing process by encouraging the application of critical thinking from assessment to evaluation.

A panel of experts put together a consensus statement in defining critical thinking as follows:

> We understand critical thinking to be purposeful, self-regulatory judgment which results in interpretation, analysis, evaluation, and inference, as well

as explanation of the evidential, conceptual, methodological, criteriological, or contextual considerations upon which that judgment is based.

(American Philosophical Association (APA) 1990)

Problem solving is goal-directed and involves evaluating the outcome of interventions so, like critical thinking, it is purposeful and involves self-regulatory judgement. For example, the nursing process and judgement are linked together in a new international classification of nursing practice (ICN 2005). The above features of critical thinking can be linked with problem solving, as follows:

Six steps to effective thinking and problem-solving
(Facione 2007: 23)

Ideals	**Five Whats and a Why**
Identify the problem	What's the real question we're facing here?
Define the context	What are the facts and circumstances that frame this problem?
Enumerate choices	What are our most plausible three or four options?
Analyse options	What is our best course of action, all things considered?
List reasons explicitly	Let's be clear: Why are we making this particular choice?
Self-correct	Okay, let's look at it again. What did we miss?

Identifying the problem and context correctly is vital, as anyone who is misdiagnosed understands, so it requires careful consideration of available evidence using appropriate assessment criteria or tools, and conceptual knowledge and understanding to make sense of (interpretation) and draw reasonable conclusions (inferences) from the information gathered. Enumerating choices and analysing options in planning actions are enhanced by reflecting on experience in dealing with such issues, awareness of pertinent policies or procedures, and critical application of relevant research evidence that is methodologically sound. This is an important stage in being able to satisfy the requirement for 'care based on the best available evidence or best practice' (NMC 2008: 7). Listing reasons to implement the chosen intervention challenges practitioners to be very clear about their rationale for using this approach and it also enables them to explain and justify decisions to others. Self-correction is the hallmark of an autonomous practitioner who is able to evaluate the strengths and weaknesses of adopted strategies in achieving desired outcomes, and, can then reassess the problem and/or consider alternative options that might be more effective in addressing it.

Effective problem solving in healthcare employs critical thinking skills, clinical judgement and decision-making in all stages of the process. Clinical judgement is defined as 'the application of information based on actual observation of a patient combined with subjective and objective data that lead to a conclusion' (Mosby 2008). It, therefore, represents a practitioner's informed opinion based on both qualitative (subjective) interpretations and quantitative (objective) analysis of observations and other relevant information sources that guide clinical decision-making. Hence, clinical judgement and decision-making are closely inter-related; the former involves assessment of alternative options whereas the latter involves choosing between alternative options (Dowie 1993).

Defining clinical decision-making

Defining clinical decision-making is important because, in doing so, the nature of healthcare itself is revealed. A valid definition of clinical decision-making in nursing must, therefore, reflect the realities of practice that nurses experience. 'Decision-making is a case of choosing between different alternatives' (Bloomsbury 2002: 408) is a simple definition highlighting a key component of decisions in committing to one course of action as opposed to others, as observed by Dowie. However, this definition is not specific to nursing and does not convey the knowledge required to determine what the available choices are, or how to review and select the most effective strategy.

Advocates of evidence-based healthcare argue that the most trustworthy source of knowledge is achieved from the results of scientific research and rigorous tests of its validity and reliability:

> Without knowledge which flows from a comprehensive and sound research and development programme, the first building block in evidence-based clinical decision-making will be missing. When such knowledge is generated it must be converted into information which is tailored to the needs of health professionals taking clinical decisions. This means focusing on the means by which evidence is made accessible and equipping staff with the skills to know how to evaluate and apply it in individual situations.
>
> (NHS Executive 1999: 8)

The promotion of research evidence-based clinical decisions to improve the quality of care is one of the aims of current NHS reforms. The National Institute for Health and Clinical Excellence (NICE) was established to conduct extensive healthcare research and produce evidence-based guidelines to inform practice. This enables local practice to benefit from a far greater accumulation of relevant information from national databases than individual practitioners' clinical experience can provide. For example, NICE guidelines for assessment and management of head injuries advise replacing skull X-rays with CT (computerized tomography) cranial scans which are far more accurate in detecting intra-cranial pathology (Hassan et al. 2005). However, it can be difficult to implement such guidelines where they depend on round-the-clock availability of specialist practitioners. In one study, of 88 patients who should have had a cranial CT scan under NICE guidelines, only ten patients did as most attended at evenings or weekends when radiologists were not at work

(Harris et al. 2006). One of the critical incidents discussed later may have had a less tragic outcome if NICE guidelines for the assessment/management of head injuries had been applied.

It is, therefore, important for nurses and other health professionals to apply relevant research in evidence-based clinical decisions but it is not always possible without additional resources. Furthermore, while it may be desirable, it is not realistic to develop research-based guidelines for every conceivable decision that nurses make. They also need to be able to process and respond to a much wider range of evidence (e.g. observations of patients, feedback, reflective practice) in addition to that provided by formal scientific research methods (Rycroft-Malone et al. 2004).

A broader and more practical understanding of clinical decision-making is conveyed in the following definition developed for nursing (but could apply to other health professions):

> Clinical decision-making is a complex process whereby practitioners determine the type of information they collect, recognize problems according to the cues identified during information collection, and decide upon appropriate interventions to address those problems.
>
> (Tanner et al. 1987)

This definition acknowledges that nurses may be able to think and act systematically to identify and address problems even when research evidence is not available to inform decisions. However, it does not convey the critical thinking skills needed or professional accountability for the decisions.

The following, more comprehensive, definition was developed in a longitudinal phenomenological study of nurses' perceptions of clinical decision-making (which is discussed later):

> Clinical decision-making is a complex process involving observation, information processing, critical thinking, evaluating evidence, applying relevant knowledge, problem solving skills, reflection and clinical judgement to select the best course of action which optimizes a patient's health and minimizes any potential harm. The role of the clinical decision-maker in nursing is, therefore, to be professionally accountable for accurately assessing patients' needs using appropriate sources of information, and planning nursing interventions that address problems and which they are competent to perform.
>
> (Standing 2005: 34)

This definition of clinical decision-making accommodates problem solving, critical thinking, judgement, scientific evidence-based practice, experiential reflective practice, ethical values and professional accountability (it could also be adapted by other health professions). It suggests that qualitative research can be valuable in portraying practitioners' perceptions of everyday reality of practice in which professional knowledge, clinical judgement and decision-making are embedded.

Normative, prescriptive, and descriptive decision-making models

According to Thompson et al. (2004) clinical decision-making models need to specify decision characteristics, information sources, decision-making processes and inter-relationships. Developing decision-making models, therefore, involves describing the types of decisions taken, identifying the knowledge and evidence required to inform decisions, critical review of methods used to process information, and understanding how all the elements are combined in clinical decision-making. Bell et al. (1995) classified decision-making models as normative, prescriptive or descriptive.

Normative models

Normative models are associated with rational, logical, scientific, evidence-based decisions informed by statistical analysis of large-scale experimental and survey research which is representative of a target population to whom the findings can be applied. Normative models are evaluated regarding their theoretical adequacy in enabling decision-makers to predict and explain the outcomes of decisions. Clinical trials that test the efficacy of new medicines and treatments are examples of this approach. Applying scientific test results also enables understanding of complex physiological processes and helps minimize judgement errors from 'base rate neglect' (Thompson 2002), for example, failing to recognize the significance of a patient's low oxygen saturation level.

Prescriptive models

Prescriptive models are associated with frameworks, guidelines or algorithms designed to enhance specific decision tasks. Prescriptive models are evaluated regarding their pragmatic adequacy in facilitating more effective decision-making. The nursing process (Yura and Walsh 1973) is an example of a prescriptive model that continues to guide systematic problem solving (ICN 2005). Prescriptive models often apply principles and findings of previous scientific research (associated with normative models), for example, in developing assessment tools and NICE clinical guidelines.

Descriptive models

Descriptive models are associated with studies that observe, describe and analyse how decisions are made by managers and professionals in relation to their day-to-day responsibilities. Descriptive models are evaluated regarding their empirical adequacy in supporting assumptions made about decision-making processes with relevant examples from a suitable period of observation. Dreyfus and Dreyfus (1980) developed a five-stage skill acquisition model in the training of United States Airforce pilots. Benner (1984) adapted Dreyfus and Dreyfus' model to describe the transition from rule-governed novice to intuitive expert nurse by eliciting practitioners' accounts of 'reflection-on-action' in tape-recorded 'phenomenological' interviews and applying the findings to support the model. The 'thinking aloud technique' where practitioners tape record what they are thinking about as they carry out actions (reflection-in-action) can also be used to develop a descriptive model of nursing and healthcare decisions (Corcoran-Perry and Narayan 1995; Schön 1983).

Applying decision-making models

Cognitive continuum theory, which combines elements of all three (normative, prescriptive, and descriptive) decision-making models, will be discussed in Chapter 5. Decision-making models and theories can be applied as educational tools: to develop conceptual understanding and relate this to practical experience; reflecting upon practice to identify professional development needs in learning and applying knowledge and skills; and practitioners mapping their experiences of clinical decision-making against decision models to help inform, analyse, explain and justify their actions. Decision theories and models can also be applied as practice guides to enhance clinical decision-making, for example, understanding how to use different evidence-based health assessment tools.

Summary of cultural influences in developing clinical decision-making skills

So far, this chapter has indicated that the clinical judgement and decision-making of nurses and/or other healthcare practitioners are subject to considerable cultural expectations from:

- **Central government** – NHS reform: reorganization, health targets, clinical governance
- **NHS trusts** – Employment contracts, appraisal, quality audit, risk management
- **Regulating bodies** – e.g. Nursing and Midwifery Council Code, professional accountability
- **Policy advisors** – NHS Service Frameworks, National Institute for Health and Clinical Excellence (NICE)
- **Educators** – Continuing professional development in evidence-based healthcare
- **Public** – Community health council, clinical governance committee, public accountability
- **Patients** – Safe, accurate and effective clinical decision-making, patient accountability.

The question then arises as to how, in light of the above influences, practitioners' clinical decision-making skills are perceived, developed, applied, and incorporated within their professional identity.

Critique of 'novice to expert' model regarding clinical judgement and decision-making

Benner's (1984) stages of skill acquisition (adapted from Dreyfus and Dreyfus) of novice, advanced beginner, competent, proficient, and expert have been widely used to portray nurses and other healthcare professionals as less reliant on rules, abstract 'calculative rationality' and analysis as they become receptive to contextual cues through experience, 'embodied knowing' and intuition. This has been helpful in suggesting how knowledge and skills are progressively, experientially integrated in developing professional identity and expertise, and in exercising clinical judgement. However, its relevance needs to be reassessed given the time that has elapsed and the many changes (referred to above) in the healthcare system that impact upon clinical decision-making. Given the importance of critical thinking in effective problem solving, clinical judgement and decision-making, criteria from the expert consensus on critical thinking (American Philosophical Association (APA) 1990) are applied to critique Benner's adaptation of the novice to expert model.

Purposeful, self-regulatory judgement (interpretation, analysis, evaluation and inference) and explanation of evidence, concepts, methods, criteria, and contexts, in 'novice to expert'

Strengths

- Purposeful, self-regulatory judgement informed by practitioners' interpretations/inferences derived from observations, interactions, and previous experience in similar clinical contexts
- Knowledge, skills and understanding embedded in and derived from practical experience which leads to the accumulation of tacit, context-sensitive, responsive, intuitive expertise.

Weaknesses

- Purposeful, self-regulatory judgement is limited where it excludes analysis and evaluation of relevant explicit scientific evidence (Benner is critical of such 'calculative rationality').
- Without analysis and evaluation it is more difficult to explain, justify and defend clinical judgements and decisions, as necessitated by public and professional accountability.
- The model is borrowed from elsewhere (how to fly a plane) and it is not sufficiently representative of the complex influences in healthcare affecting clinical judgement and decision-making.
- Nurses' interview responses were used to support application of 'novice to expert' model in nursing which is inconsistent with phenomenological principles and the methods described.

- Instead of interviewing the same nurses over a long period to demonstrate their transition from 'novice to expert', different nurses were used at each interview stage to save time.

In summary, Benner's adaptation of the 'novice to expert' model is biased in favour of intuition and against analysis, which is at odds with the new culture of scientific evidence-based healthcare and the principle of open-minded, critical thinking 'honest in facing personal biases' (APA 1990: 22). Despite Benner championing experiential and contextual understanding, the model derives from a completely different occupational context and nurses' responses are used to support it (a bit too neatly) rather than developing new concepts derived from nurses' unique 'lived experience'. The matrix model, which follows, offers an alternative which addresses many of the above criticisms.

Perceptions of clinical decision-making – a matrix model

A matrix model of clinical decision-making was developed during a longitudinal study (2000–2004) recording the developmental journey of the same respondents throughout their pre-registration nursing programme and first year as registered nurses (Standing 2005, 2007). Its timing coincided with NHS and educational reforms, discussed earlier, and its phenomenological methods focused on eliciting and understanding respondents' 'lived experience' in acquiring and applying clinical decision-making skills, including coping with their responsibilities as first year staff nurses. A series of in-depth, tape-recorded interviews were the main source of data collection that explored:

- Conceptions of nursing
- Perceptions of clinical decision-making
- Personal, theoretical, and practice influences upon clinical decision-making skills
- Critical incident analysis of clinical decision-making as registered nurses.

Conceptions of nursing were included to explore respondents' understanding of professional identity and to compare this with their perceptions of clinical decision-making as they gained experience and took on more responsibility. The interviews were timed to coincide with significant milestones that provided a context to explore respondents' experience and 'reflection-on-action':

1. 3–5 months   After completing introduction to programme
2. 18–20 months   After completing common foundation
3. 32–34 months   Before completing Adult/Mental Health/
                     Child Branch
4. 42–48 months   After completing preceptorship as newly registered
                     nurses

In addition, respondents kept reflective diaries of their experiences, achievements and challenges throughout the study and referred to these during interviews to reduce problems of recall. They were also given transcripts to check and shown examples of how their extracts had contributed to the thematic analysis of interview data. Hence, respondents acted as co-researchers to document experiences, create inter-subjective understanding during interviews, and to validate the accounts, analysis and co-constituted (agreed) meaning of their lived clinical experience (Drauker 1999). The sample (n = 20) was reasonably representative of the student cohort (n = 134) from which it was taken in terms of education, age range, gender, ethnicity, and nursing branch preference.

Identifying 'conceptions of nursing' themes from interview transcripts

Respondents were asked about their personal history, why they wanted to be nurses, and their views on the role, attributes and qualities needed. Ten conceptions of nursing were identified:

Conceptions of nursing	Related terms used
Caring:	Cheer people up, supportive, helping through tough time, friendly
Listening and being there:	You need patient to express what they feel, spending time with
Practical procedures:	Hands-on care, assessments, bandaging, injections, life saver.
Knowledge and understanding:	Clued up, holistic, infection control, analysing, constantly evaluating.
Communicating:	Talking to patients, giving information or advice, acting as advocate.
Patience:	Tolerance, right temperament, you have to have a fairly long fuse
Teamwork:	Bridge between patient and doctor, gain trust of other staff
Paperwork:	Record observations, administration, planning care, medical history
Empathizing/ Non-judgemental:	Not judging or making their worries seem insignificant, have respect
Professional:	Know boundaries; manage emotions, conscientious, competent.

All of the themes were identified in Interview 1. The respondents were also asked to describe their conceptions of nursing in Interviews 2–4. Their responses confirmed themes previously identified with a particular emphasis on mastering practical procedures, developing greater knowledge and understanding, valuing teamwork as source of support, and a growing awareness of responsibility in becoming a professional nurse. Their apparent broad understanding of nursing so early in the programme was associated with previous healthcare experience, a high proportion of mature entrants, caring for children as parents, and long-standing motivation e.g. family history of nursing.

Reflective activity 1.1

Imagine you are asked to prepare an hour-long talk describing your own health-care profession to a group of school leavers:

1. Write down the first things that spring to mind in describing your role and the attributes and personal qualities needed to perform it.
2. Think about your own reasons for becoming a nurse (or other healthcare professional) and make notes about what the profession currently has to offer new potential recruits.
3. If you are a nurse, write down the above list of conceptions of nursing, then go through each one and identify examples showing how they relate to your own area of practice. If you are not a nurse, devise your own list of conceptions and give examples of each one.
4. Ask one or two colleagues to do the same activity and then arrange to meet up, compare notes regarding responses to steps 1–3, and amend lists if desired.
5. Reflect upon whether or not you think the true nature of professional identity has been revealed. Is there anything you want to add? Do you feel able to explain it to others?

Identifying 'perceptions of clinical decision-making' themes from interview transcripts

In Interview 1 respondents were asked how they made decisions using examples from family or social life and work experience. In Interview 2 they reflected on their observations of a 'typical day' in practice placements regarding contact with patients, tasks involved in, choices made, and what they learned about clinical decision-making. In Interview 3 they described examples of how they had contributed to planning patient care and were prompted to explain and justify their rationale. In Interview 4 they engaged in critical incident analysis of their clinical decision-making experiences as newly registered nurses. Ten perceptions of clinical decision-making were identified.

Perceptions of clinical decision-making	Examples
Collaborative:	Discuss care with patients/relatives, colleagues, other professionals
Experience (and intuition):	Previous similar cases inform actions (and 'unconscious' assessment')
Confidence:	Less self-conscious, can justify decision, able to perform tasks safely
Systematic:	Assess, plan, implement and evaluate care, logical, critical thinker

Prioritizing: Organize care re: emergencies, patient dependency, health targets

Observation: Respond to patients' vital signs, appearance, 'read' body language

Standardized: Apply policies, assessment tools, procedural guidelines, care plans

Reflective: Think about experience, learn from it; work out what to do differently

Ethical sensitivity: Break 'bad news' compassionately, dealing with treatment dilemmas

Accountability: Explain actions to patients, report mistakes, law e.g. Child Protection

The first five themes in the list were identified in Interview 1 (except that 'intuition' was added to 'experience' in Interview 4). The other five themes were identified in Interview 2. All of the themes were applicable in subsequent interviews and no new ones were needed to explain additional data. Collectively the themes summarize respondents' four-year developmental journey in acquiring and applying clinical decision-making skills from novice students to competent registered nurses. In doing so they convey awareness and response to cultural influences associated with NHS reforms, health targets, public accountability, evidence-based decisions, enhancing the quality of patients' experience and outcomes of care, and effective organization and collaboration in delivering care. The themes also offer support for Standing's definition of clinical decision-making described earlier.

Reflective activity 1.2

Imagine you are asked to do a one-hour talk to a group of third year students about the application of clinical judgement and decision-making skills in your area of healthcare practice.

1. Write down the first things that spring to mind in describing the clinical decisions you have to make and the way you go about making a decision.
2. Reflect upon how your understanding of clinical judgement and decision-making has developed since you were a student and write down what has helped and/or guided you.
3. Write down the list of perceptions of clinical decision-making, identify examples for each of the themes relating them to your own clinical practice, and then add them to your list.
4. Ask one or two colleagues to do the same activity and then arrange to meet up, compare notes regarding responses to steps 1–3, and amend lists if desired.
5. Reflect upon whether or not you think the true nature of clinical decision-making has been revealed. Is there anything you want to add? Do you feel able to explain it to others?

Matrix combining conceptions of nursing and perceptions of clinical decision-making

So far, ten conceptions of nursing and ten perceptions of clinical decision-making have been listed separately, but professional identity and clinical judgement/decision-making are closely linked, as indicated in the RCN definition of nursing (2003). (Readers who are not nurses could substitute their own profession where nursing is referred to as the principles are transferable.) Miles and Huberman (1994) described how matrices are useful to organize and present different categories of data, so to show how respondents' accounts linked the two thematic categories a matrix was generated for each set of interview data. Therefore, the matrix model is made up of a series of four matrices that cross-reference perceptions of clinical decision-making with conceptions of nursing, highlighting any inter-relationships over a four-year developmental journey from novice nursing students to competent registered nurses (Standing 2005, 2007). If information in a transcript extract supports both a perception of clinical decision-making and a conception of nursing then an inter-relationship is recorded on the matrix. Figure 1.1 cross-references perceptions of clinical decision-making and conceptions of nursing in Interview 1: 3–5 months (novice nursing students):

In Figure 1.1, 20 respondents revealed five inter-relationships (out of a potential 50) between perceptions of clinical decision-making (upper case) and conceptions of nursing, as follows:

A. **COLLABORATIVE/Teamwork:** Choosing different members of the team to approach according to the nature of the decision and who you think would be best suited to advise you.
B. **EXPERIENCE/Knowledge and understanding:** Mistaken for a staff nurse (mufti worn) by students on placement due to ability to teach them about both patient care and role/function of the unit.
C. **CONFIDENCE/Teamwork:** Healthcare assistant working alone at night worried about elderly patient summoned night supervisor, problem resolved, felt satisfied it was right to call for help.
D. **SYSTEMATIC/Listening and being there:** Listened to children's fear of flying, went by boat, next year took them to watch planes taking off/landing several times, eased concerns before flight.
E. **PRIORITIZING/Knowledge and understanding:** Understanding some patients are more dependent and less able to help themselves than others, and making their care a priority.

All of these examples referred to respondents' experience before starting the nursing programme and most relate to healthcare assistant work. Even novice students may have previous life experiences which are relevant to clinical judgement and decision-making in their chosen healthcare profession. Although the 'systematic' example was about a family holiday it was included because the skills of listening to anxieties, changing plans, devising and implementing an action plan to reduce children's fear, are transferable to clinical

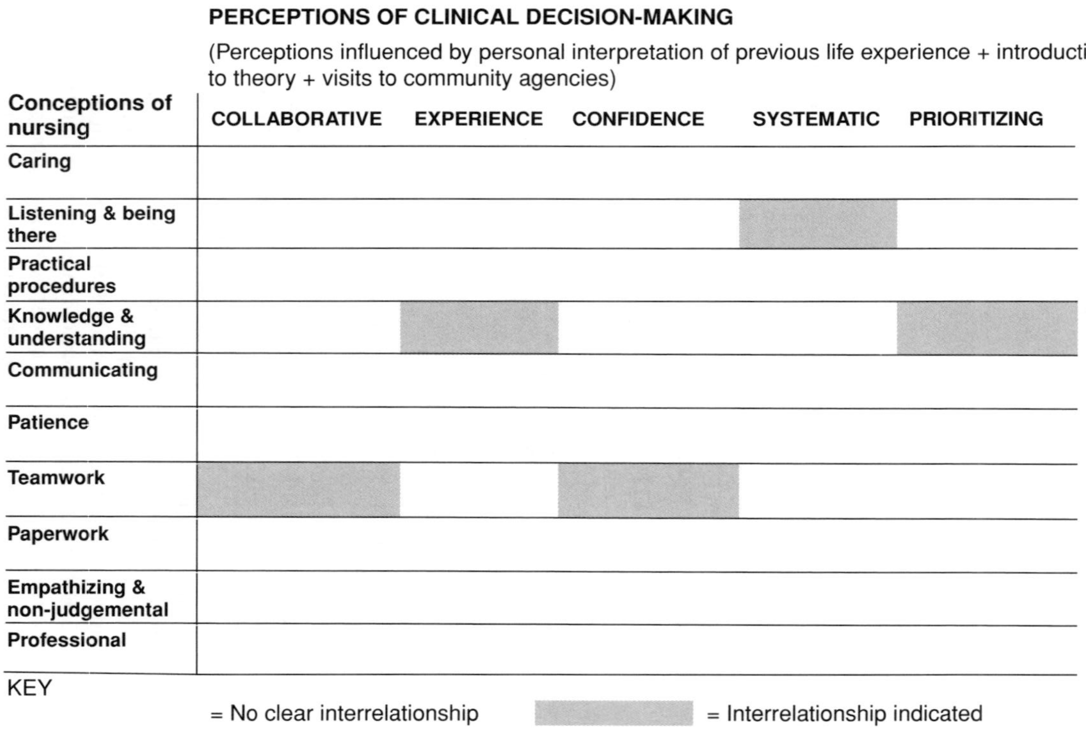

PERCEPTIONS OF CLINICAL DECISION-MAKING

(Perceptions influenced by personal interpretation of previous life experience + introduction to theory + visits to community agencies)

Conceptions of nursing	COLLABORATIVE	EXPERIENCE	CONFIDENCE	SYSTEMATIC	PRIORITIZING
Caring					
Listening & being there				▓	
Practical procedures					
Knowledge & understanding		▓			▓
Communicating					
Patience					
Teamwork	▓		▓		
Paperwork					
Empathizing & non-judgemental					
Professional					

KEY

= No clear interrelationship   ▓ = Interrelationship indicated

Figure 1.1 Matrix 1: Perceptions of clinical decision-making/conceptions of nursing after 3–5 months as nursing students (n = 20) (Standing 2005, 2007)

decision-making (especially given that this respondent elected to specialize in children's nursing). The small proportion of inter-relationships reflects the timing of interviews and a disparity between respondents' conceptual understanding of nursing and their actual experience of clinical decision-making. Figure 1.2 shows a considerable increase in inter-relationships between perceptions of clinical decision-making and conceptions of nursing themes by Interview 4: 42–48 months (after 6–12 months as staff nurses):

In Figure 1.2 ten respondents revealed 65 inter-relationships (out of a potential 100) between clinical decision-making (upper case) and conceptions of nursing themes by reflecting on critical incidents with a 'discernible impact' (Polit and Hungler 1999: 332) on them, as they came to terms with a wide range of clinical decision-making responsibilities as registered nurses. For example:

A. **COLLABORATIVE/Teamwork:** Dealing with an emergency on ward when received phone call that one of our patients had collapsed elsewhere in hospital, asked nurses from next ward for help, they stabilized him, we discovered he had a problem that was missed during assessment.

B. **EXPERIENCE and INTUITION/Professional:** Refused to give prescribed injection to child in A&E who was fitting, did not feel competent, unfamiliar drug so corrosive it needed a glass syringe, doctor gave injection, read up on drug and would give it next time. Felt I made right decision.

C. **CONFIDENCE/Communicating:** First patient cared for after qualifying was depressed, always lying on bed not interacting with anyone, primary nurse busy, so I talked to him, engaged him in planning care, addressed dietary issues, mood lifted, discharged home. I felt I had contributed.

D. **SYSTEMATIC/Knowledge and understanding:** A lady shouted her baby had turned blue, I was on my own, had no experience of this but remembered lesson from nurse tutor, recognized signs of severe respiratory distress, airway was obstructed, cleared obstruction and revived the baby.

E. **PRIORITIZING/Teamwork:** Patient very pale, sweating, complaining of chest pain and terrible indigestion, suspected M.I. (myocardial infarction), asked colleague to call 'Crash' team, then patient in next bed said her chest hurt, so asked what pain was like, I knew it was not her heart.

F. **OBSERVATION/Knowledge and understanding:** Assessing A&E patient with history of slow onset weakness, confusion. I suspected TIA (trans-ischaemic attack). Then pupils 'blew', he vomited, transferred to 'Resus', but died two hours later. Discovered from wife he bumped head in car accident day before, had skull X-ray (different hospital), did not show anything wrong so was sent home. Angry with self for missing head injury/vowed to get more accurate history in future.

G. **STANDARDIZED/Practical procedures:** Procedure for intravenous infusion stipulates use of an automatic pump but they were all being used, set flow rate manually instead, flow rate sped up, went through

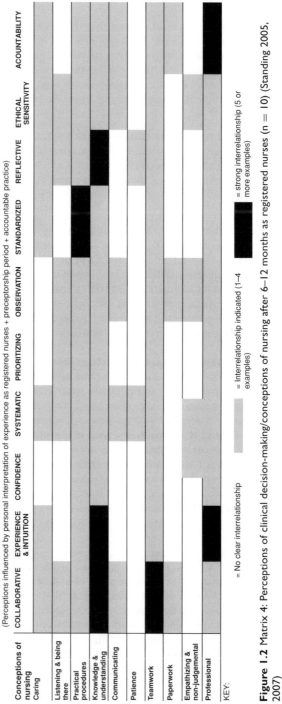

Figure 1.2 Matrix 4: Perceptions of clinical decision-making/conceptions of nursing after 6–12 months as registered nurses (n = 10) (Standing 2005, 2007)

too fast, had to fill in 'incident form', should have got pump from site coordinator.

H. **REFLECTIVE/Knowledge and understanding:** Patient with history of drug misuse asked for PRN (pro re nata – to be given at nurses' discretion) medication every day. It was addictive, worried I might be encouraging misuse so I asked him why he needed it, sometimes he just smiled so I didn't give it; if he gave valid reason for being stressed I did give it – always reviewing decision.

I. **ETHICAL SENSITIVITY/Caring:** Elderly patient (98), no living relatives, not eating or drinking enough and refusing alternatives. Dilemma: without intravenous fluid/nutrients she might die quite soon; with them she would live longer but we would be denying her right to choose. Team agreed to respect her wishes but to continue offering food and drink, and someone to talk to.

J. **ACCOUNTABILITY/Professional:** Gave intravenous antibiotic to patient, phone rang, asked me to say he could not talk, forgot to sign drug chart resulting in later shift giving an extra dose, had to report to matron, explain mistake to patient and consultant, will finish task first in future.

The nurses described their role transition as registered nurses (6–12 months) as a 'steep learning curve' in which they had to 'think on their feet' without the 'comfort blanket' of student status. The strong 'Collaborative', 'Experience and Intuition', 'Standardized', 'Reflective', and 'Accountability' perceptions in Figure 1.2 show a heightened awareness of: joint decision-making; value of practical experience; approved way to do procedures; ongoing review of actions; and professional status and responsibilities. Six critical incidents involved the nurses intervening in life-threatening situations (A, B, D, E, F, I) and in one case (F) the patient died. In four critical incidents they had to resolve dilemmas (A, B, H, I) in deciding what to do when: simultaneous emergencies occur and you cannot manage both; a child urgently needs an injection but you do not feel competent to give it; a patient who misused drugs requests discretionary medication and you're not sure he needs it; an elderly patient declines food and drink and will not consent to intravenous fluids or supplements.

The urgency and complexity of healthcare problems described highlight the challenging nature of clinical judgement and decision-making in nursing, and the potential risks if mistakes are made.

Three critical incidents involved errors of judgement (F, G, J) that are linked to non-compliance with 'Standardized' procedures. If head injury patient (F) had been managed according to NICE guidelines at the first hospital he would have had a cranial CT scan and might still be alive as it is more likely an intra-cranial haemorrhage would have been detected and treated. Head injuries account for 10–20 per cent of all emergency department admissions (Hassan et al. 2005) so in patients with neurological symptoms the proportion of head injuries is much higher. Not knowing the history, the nurse made a plausible provisional diagnosis that excluded head injury. This type of mistake is an example of 'anchoring bias' and 'base rate neglect' (Thompson 2002) that disregards relevant head injury incidence and morbidity. In incident G the problem arose due to a lack of 'Standardized' equipment (automatic pump) for the procedure. The flow rate speeding up without the nurse noticing (distracted looking after other A&E patients) is an example of 'interference error' which is prevented by more frequent 'Observation'. In incident J, giving injection, answering patient's phone, forgetting to sign drug chart is an example of 'omission following interruption' (Thompson 2002). The incidents (F, G, J) had a profound effect on the nurses' understanding of their 'Accountability' for clinical decisions, and they were 'Reflective' about feelings/ thoughts/actions in learning how to avoid such mistakes in future.

All of the registered nurses' clinical decisions (including errors) can be understood in relation to the ten identified perceptions of clinical decision-making in the matrix model. The summaries of critical incidents (A–J) show each perception individually applied to one aspect of different situations. This helps clarify distinctions between them but in practice each situation involved applying many of the perceptions collectively. The growing pattern of inter-relationships between clinical decision-making and conceptions of nursing themes corresponds with the respondents' transition from novice nursing students to competent registered nurses. They associated their development as nurses with personal influences (e.g. maturing), theoretical influences (e.g. research awareness), and practice influences (e.g. accountability for care delivery). This supports the view that 'Professional practice requires knowledge derived from research and theory, from professional practice, and from personal experience' (Higgs and Titchen 2001: 4–5). The matrix model helps to explain how practitioners make sense of and integrate personal understanding, theoretical and experiential knowledge, and their practical experience of acquiring and applying clinical decision-making skills.

Reflective activity 1.3

Refer back to the examples you were asked to identify in Reflective activities 1.1 and 1.2.

1. Look at each conception of nursing/healthcare profession example and identify one or more perceptions of clinical decision-making that you associate with it and explain why.
2. Look at each perception of clinical decision-making example and identify one or more conception of nursing/healthcare profession that you associate with it and explain why.
3. Draw a matrix grid identifying the perceptions of clinical decision-making on one axis and conceptions of nursing/health profession themes on the other axis.

4. Refer to information generated in steps 1 and 2 and plot inter-relationships between perceptions of clinical decision-making and conceptions of nursing/healthcare profession on matrix grid.
5. Do you notice a pattern? How much interaction is there between perceptions of clinical decision-making and conceptions of nursing/healthcare profession? Does the matrix enable you to relate clinical decision-making processes to your own sense of professional identity?
6. Consider how you might apply the matrix model to describe and reflect upon your own clinical decision-making and in identifying any ongoing professional development needs.

Critique of the matrix model of clinical decision-making

Decision theory (Bell et al. 1995; Thompson et al. 2004) and critical thinking criteria (APA 1990) referred to earlier are applied to evaluate the strengths, weaknesses and relevance of the matrix model of clinical decision-making in nursing and healthcare.

Is the matrix a normative, prescriptive or descriptive decision-making model?

The matrix model is based on a relatively small-scale qualitative (phenomenological) study so it is not a normative model. However, the 'Standardized' theme incorporates normative features, for example, nurses referred to having 'to know the normal ranges of blood' when reviewing test results, and using research-based guidelines such as an 'inventory of suicidal intention' when assessing risks associated with caring for a depressed patient. The matrix model is not prescriptive as it seeks to explain how nurses perceive clinical decision-making rather than give advice on what to do, and it does not advocate a preference for any particular style of decision-making. However, the 'Systematic' theme incorporates prescriptive features, for example, nurses referred to applying the nursing process to assess, diagnose, plan, implement and evaluate care. The matrix is a descriptive model informed by nurses' 'reflection-on-action', describing their experience and understanding of clinical decision-making, during in-depth audio-taped interviews. Each clinical decision-making theme is supported by transcript extracts which attest to its empirical adequacy.

Matrix model decision characteristics, information sources, processes, and inter-relationships

Qualitative studies, such as the one from which the matrix model is derived, may be criticized for being too localized and having such small samples that generalizing findings to a wider population is not viable. A good test of the matrix model's relevance is to compare it with a large-scale survey of nurses' research information use and classification of nursing decisions (Cullum 2002):

Comparison of decision characteristics

Matrix model	Survey nurses' information use
(Standing 2005)	(Cullum 2002)
Practical procedures	Intervention/effectiveness
PRIORITIZING/Patience	Targeting and timing
Communicating	Communication
COLLABORATIVE/Teamwork/	Service organization, delivery and
Paperwork	management
EXPERIENCE and INTUITION	Experiential, understanding or
	hermeneutic
ETHICAL SENSITIVITY	
ACCOUNTABILITY	

As illustrated above, all of the broad categories of decision characteristics identified in Cullum's large survey are represented in the matrix model. In addition, the matrix model identifies 'Ethical sensitivity' and 'Accountability' which, as NHS reforms emphasize and the above extracts indicate, are also significant factors influencing decisions. This indicates that the findings of an in-depth qualitative study, summarized in the matrix model, are supported by and add to the findings of a larger quantitative study. The matrix model appears relevant, topical and representative of the wide variety of clinical decision characteristics associated with nurses more generally.

Matrix model information sources include 'Knowledge and understanding' (personal, theoretical, experiential, and practical), 'Observation', 'Listening and being there', and 'Confidence' (trust in evidence). In this way the matrix model balances formal/explicit and informal/tacit knowledge and skills that inform clinical judgement and decision-making (Eraut 2000; Gabbay and le May 2004).

Matrix model clinical decision-making processes synthesize contrasting styles: 'Standardized' and 'Systematic' themes relate to evidence-based practice or 'technical/calculative rationality', while 'Collaborative' and 'Reflective' themes relate to reflective practice and 'professional/embodied knowing' (Schön 1983; Benner 1984). In addition, 'Caring', 'Empathizing and non-judgemental', and 'Professional' themes convey an awareness that clinical judgement, decision-making and nursing interventions must be in patients' best interests and of a high standard (NMC 2008).

Inter-relationships define the structure of the matrix model where conceptions of nursing are cross-referenced with perceptions of decision-making. Snyder (1995: 33) says a 'conceptual model used by a nurse provides the basis for making the complex decisions that are crucial in the delivery of good nursing care'. However, nurses may not usually be aware of their personal, tacit 'mental models' and how these influence behaviour (Krejci 1997). Rather than impose a theoretical framework to analyse respondents' experience, their experience produced the themes that were applied and revised to interpret their continuing development. Therefore, the matrix model collates and articulates nurses' understanding and experience of: a wide range of decisions; evidence referred to; clinical decision-making strategies used; and professional values they associate with nursing.

Purposeful, self-regulatory judgement (interpretation, analysis, evaluation and inference) and explanation of evidence, concepts, methods, criteria, and contexts, in the matrix model

Strengths

- Purposeful, self-regulatory judgement informed by practitioners' interpretations/inferences derived from observations, interactions, and previous experience in similar clinical contexts, plus systematic problem solving, analysis and evaluation of relevant scientific evidence.
- Knowledge, skills and understanding are embedded in and derived from practical experience which leads to the accumulation of tacit, context-sensitive, responsive, intuitive expertise. It is also explicit, evidence-based, applying relevant research findings from wider population.
- The criteria of conceptions of nursing/healthcare and clinical decision-making perceptions enable practitioners' understanding, acquisition and application of decision-making skills to be described and continually related to the development of their professional identity.
- The concepts/themes identified in the matrix model are derived from research evidence of extensive verbatim transcript extracts and are also supported by current relevant literature.
- A new comprehensive definition of clinical decision-making in nursing (which could be adapted by other health professions) was developed from the matrix model (see page 7).
- Phenomenological (hermeneutic) methods ensured credibility of the findings via repeated in-depth interviews of the same respondents over four years, reflecting upon the knowledge embedded in the 'average everydayness' (Heidegger 1962: 38) of their clinical practice.
- A new critical framework was developed (Standing 2005, 2009) to critique trustworthiness and rigour of the research study on which the matrix model is based by synthesizing phenomenological and qualitative evaluation criteria (Lincoln and Guba 1985; Sandelowski 1986; Annells 1999) with hermeneutic concepts and existential philosophy (Heidegger 1962).

Weaknesses

- Dependence on self-reports (retrospective reflection-on-action) has been criticized as a less reliable form of evidence than direct observation of clinical practice (Thompson et al. 2004). However, there are ethical and practical difficulties in direct observation of patient contact.

- There was a high attrition rate as only ten of the original 20 respondents remained at the final interview. This is not uncommon in longitudinal studies (Murphy-Black 2000).
- The matrix is not a normative or prescriptive decision model so it is limited in advising what, how, or why decisions should be made. As a descriptive model it is useful in representing, explaining and raising practitioners' awareness of their clinical decision-making skills.

Summary

This chapter has indicated that nurses and other health professionals are subject to considerable cultural pressure from government, health service providers, regulators, advisors, educators, the public, and patients in their care to demonstrate safe and effective clinical decision-making skills. Clinical decision-making was described as the product of clinical judgement and critical thinking skills applied to problem solving within healthcare settings. Analytical scientific, evidence-based and intuitive reflective, experiential processes of clinical judgement and decision-making were discussed in relation to normative, prescriptive and descriptive decision models and professional identity in healthcare. Benner's 'novice to expert' model was considered to be biased in favour of intuition and against analysis, and an alternative matrix model, derived from an in-depth longitudinal study of nurses' development of clinical decision-making skills, was presented. This revealed that registered nurses are responsible for a wide range of challenging decisions affecting the well-being and survival of patients, using various information sources, combining both evidence-based and reflective decision-making processes within ethical, accountable nursing practice. A definition was developed to reflect the complexity of clinical decision-making in nursing/healthcare. A critique of the matrix indicated it is a relevant descriptive model of clinical decision-making skills. Reflective activities were suggested to enable readers to apply the matrix model and associated research findings to their own healthcare experience and to identify professional development needs.

Key points

- Professional identity is embedded within healthcare practitioners' clinical judgement/decision-making and related care patients receive.
- NHS reform, reorganization and clinical governance require greater scrutiny and public accountability of healthcare practitioners' clinical decision-making skills.
- Clinical judgement is informed opinion about available options; decision-making is choosing an option in order to take action; and, both apply critical thinking to problem solving in healthcare.

- Nursing (e.g. caring), and decision-making (e.g. collaborative, systematic, standardized, reflective) themes, summarized in a matrix model, were derived from nurses' reflections.
- The matrix model combines elements of reflective practice, evidence-based practice, ethical sensitivity, professional accountability, and personal/practical/ theoretical knowledge and skills.
- Decision errors from inattentiveness or restricted focus (anchoring bias) were linked with non-compliance to guidelines, high workload and lack of equipment/ services, e.g. no '24/7' CT scan.
- Registered nurses have to 'think on their feet' to cope with a high volume/intensity of constantly changing clinical demands, including life-threatening emergencies and ethical dilemmas.

References

American Philosophical Association (APA) (1990) *Critical Thinking: A statement of expert consensus*. The Delphi Report. Committee on Pre-College Philosophy. ERIC Doc. No. ED 315, 423.

Annells, M. (1999) Evaluating phenomenology: usefulness, quality and philosophical foundations. *Nurse Researcher*, 6(3): 5–19.

Bell, D.E., Raiffa, H. and Tversky, A. (1995) Descriptive, normative and prescriptive interactions in decision making, in D.E. Bell, H. Raiffa and A. Tversky (eds) *Decision Making*. Cambridge: Cambridge University Press.

Benner, P. (1984) *From Novice to Expert*. Menlo Park, CA: Addison-Wesley.

Benner, P., Tanner, C.A. and Chesla, C.A. (1996) *Expertise in Nursing Practice: Caring, clinical judgement and ethics*. New York: Springer.

Bloomsbury (2002) *Business: The ultimate resource*. London: Bloomsbury Publications.

Corcoran-Perry, S. and Narayan, S. (1995) Clinical decision making, in M. Snyder and M.P. Mirr (eds) *Advanced Nursing Practice*. New York: Springer.

Cullum, N. (2002) *Nurses' Use of Research Information in Clinical Decision Making: A descriptive and analytical study*. London: DH.

Department of Health (1998) *A First Class Service: Quality in the new NHS*. London: DH.

Department of Health (1999) *Agenda for Change: Modernising the NHS pay system*. London: DH.

Department of Health (2000) *The NHS Plan: A plan for investment, a plan for reform*. London: DH.

Department of Health (2001) *Working Together, Learning Together: A framework for lifelong learning for the NHS*. London: DH.

Dowding, D. and Thompson, C. (2002) Decision making and judgements in nursing: some conclusions, in C. Thompson and D. Dowding (eds) *Clinical Decision Making and Judgement in Nursing*. Edinburgh: Churchill Livingstone.

Dowie, J. (1993) Clinical decision analysis: background and introduction, in H. Llewelyn and A. Hopkins (eds) *Analysing How We Reach Clinical Decisions*. London: Royal College of Physicians.

Drauker, C.B. (1999) The critique of Heideggerian hermeneutic nursing research. *Journal of Advanced Nursing*, 30(2): 360–73.

Dreyfus, S.E. and Dreyfus, H.L. (1980) *A Five Stage Model of the Mental Activities Involved in Directed Skill Acquisition*. Operations Research Centre, 80–82. Berkeley: University of California.

Eraut, M. (2000) Non-formal learning and tacit knowledge in professional work. *British Journal of Educational Psychology,* 70: 113–16.

Facione, P.A. (2007) *Critical Thinking: What it is and why it counts.* Millbrae, CA: California Academic Press.

Gabbay, J. and le May, A. (2004) Evidence based guidelines or collectively constructed 'mindlines?'. Ethnographic study of knowledge management in primary care. *British Medical Journal,* 329(7473): 1013–19.

Gonzalez, J. and Wagenaar, R. (eds) (2005) *Tuning Educational Structures in Europe: Final Report Pilot Project – Phase 2.* Bilbao: University of Deusto.

Harris, A., Williams, D., Jain, N. and Lockey, A. (2006) Management of minor head injuries according to NICE guidelines and changes in the number of patients requiring computerised tomography imaging in a district general hospital. *International Journal of Clinical Practice,* 60(9): 1120–2.

Hassan, Z., Smith, M., Littlewood, S. et al. (2005) Head injuries: a study evaluating the impact of the NICE head injury guidelines. *Emergency Medical Journal,* 22: 845–9.

Heidegger, M. (1962) *Being and Time.* Translated by J. Macquarrie and E. Robinson. New York: Harper Row.

Henderson, V. (1966) *The Nature of Nursing.* New York: Macmillan.

Higgs, J. and Titchen, A. (2001) *Practice Knowledge and Expertise.* Oxford: Butterworth Heinemann.

Hurst, K., Dean, A. and Trickery, S. (1991) The recognition and non recognition of problem solving strategies in nursing practice. *Journal of Advanced Nursing,* 16: 1444–55.

International Council of Nurses (ICN) (2005) *International Classification of Nursing Practice [ICNP] Version 1.0 Book Chapter 4 – The 7-Axis Model.* Geneva: ICN. http://www.icn.ch/icnp_v1book_ch4.htm (accessed 5 January 2007).

Krejci, J.W. (1997) Imagery: stimulating critical thinking by exploring mental models. *Journal of Nursing Education,* 36(10): 482–4.

Lincoln, Y.S. and Guba, E. (1985) *Naturalistic Enquiry.* Beverly Hills: Sage.

Miles, M.B. and Huberman, A.M. (1994) *Qualitative Data Analysis.* Thousand Oaks, CA: Sage.

Mosby (2008) *Mosby's Medical Dictionary,* 8th edn. St. Louis, MO: Mosby.

Murphy-Black, T. (2000) Longitudinal research, in D. Cormack (ed.) *The Research Process in Nursing,* 4th edn. Oxford: Blackwell Science.

National Health Service (NHS) Executive (1999) *Clinical Governance: Quality in the new NHS.* Leeds: NHS Executive.

Nursing and Midwifery Council (NMC) (2004) *Standards of Proficiency for Pre-registration Nursing Education.* London: NMC.

Nursing and Midwifery Council (NMC) (2008) *The Code: Standards of conduct, performance and ethics for nurses and midwives.* London: NMC.

Parse, R.R. (1981) *Man-living-health: A theory of nursing.* New York: Wiley.

Pilkington, F.B. (2005) The concept of intentionality in human science nursing theories. *Nursing Science Quarterly,* 18(2): 98–104.

Polit, D.F. and Hungler, B.P. (1999) *Nursing Research: Principles and methods.* Philadelphia: Lippincott.

Royal College of Nursing (RCN) (2003) *Defining Nursing.* London: RCN.

Rycroft-Malone, J., Seers, K., Titchen, A. Harvey, G., Kitson, A. and McCormack, B. (2004) What counts as evidence-based practice? *Journal of Advanced Nursing,* 47(1): 81–90.

Sandelowski, M. (1986) The problem of rigor in qualitative research. *Advances in Nursing Science,* 8(3): 27–37.

Schön, D.A. (1983) *The Reflective Practitioner.* New York: Basic Books.

Snyder, M. (1995) Advance practice within a nursing paradigm, in M. Snyder and M.P. Mirr (eds) *Advanced Nursing Practice.* New York: Springer.

Standing, M. (2005) Perceptions of clinical decision-making on a developmental journey from student to staff nurse. PhD thesis, Canterbury, University of Kent.

Standing, M. (2007) Clinical decision-making skills on the developmental journey from student to registered nurse: a longitudinal inquiry. *Journal of Advanced Nursing,* 60(3): 257–69.

Standing, M. (2009) A new critical framework for applying hermeneutic phenomenology. *Nurse Researcher,* 16(4): 20–30.

Tanner, C.A., Padrick, K., Westfall, U.E. and Putzier, D.J. (1987) Diagnostic reasoning strategies of nurses and nursing students. *Nursing Research,* 36(6): 358–63.

Thompson, C. (2002) Human error, bias, decision making and judgement in nursing: the need for a systematic approach, in C. Thompson and D. Dowding (eds) *Clinical Decision Making and Judgement in Nursing.* Edinburgh: Churchill Livingstone.

Thompson, C. et al. (2004) Nurses, information use, and clinical making – the real world potential for evidence-based decisions in nursing, *Evidence-based Nursing,* 7: 68–72.

United Kingdom Central Council (UKCC) (1999) *Fitness for Practice.* London: UKCC.

United Kingdom Central Council (UKCC) (2001) *Fitness for Practice and Purpose.* London: UKCC.

Yura, H. and Walsh, M.B. (1973) *The Nursing Process: Assessing, planning, implementing, evaluating,* 2nd edn. New York: Appleton-Century-Crofts.

2 Advanced practitioners and advanced practice

Kate Dewar

Overview

In this chapter, the individual attributes that characterize the effective advanced practitioner are discussed in terms of their relevance to advanced practice decision-making. The different 'levels of practice' in UK healthcare are examined in relation to their historical development and subsequent implications for advanced practice. Significant elements that typify the advanced level of practice are examined, in order to identify and clarify the scope of advanced practice decision-making.

Objectives

- Describe the blend of personal characteristics that advanced practitioners require in order to effectively carry out their care/service improvement functions
- Identify the discriminating features of advanced and consultant levels of practice
- Understand the differences between generic, common, shared and specific competences
- Describe advanced practitioner roles with reference to career framework descriptors
- Recognize how personal characteristics and role requirements influence one's own decision-making expertise

Advanced practitioners and their working environment

The Skills for Health organization (2009) describes advanced practitioners as:

> experienced clinical professionals who have developed their skills and theoretical knowledge to a very high standard. They are empowered to make high-level clinical decisions and will often have their own caseload. Non-clinical staff... will typically be managing a number of service areas.

The UK Government supports the introduction of advanced practitioner roles, but only if they bring about practice or service improvements (DH 1999). Thus, these practitioners must function as innovators/entrepreneurs within their organization. In order to operate in this way, they must carry out sophisticated decision-related processes when performing their role functions (DH 1997; NES 2007).

Innovators, or entrepreneurs, are most effective when they work in a culture of entrepreneurialism (Littunen 2000). The entrepreneurial organization is one that constantly monitors itself for the presence of innovative practices which will move the organization forward, towards its improvement goals. In this evaluation process, any goals/targets reached are perceived as intermediate not end points, so that innovative practices are always taking place (Thompson 1999). Consequently, advanced practice entrepreneurs can only fully contribute to the improvement of practice, using their decision-making expertise, if the organizational structure and culture support entrepreneurship. For example, Fuller and Warren (2006) suggest that innovating and changing practice in a continuous, cyclical way occurs most effectively by utilizing stakeholder-group reflexive processes, because opportunities for entrepreneurs to have practice/service improvement insights are multiplied when ideas are shared. Therefore, in order to facilitate entrepreneurial activities, the organization should be structured, at all its levels, to facilitate the sharing of stakeholders' ideas about current problems and potential solutions.

Personal characteristics of advanced practitioners

Literature suggests that it is the personal characteristics of advanced practitioners which determine whether they can achieve the level of decision-making ability required at their level of practice (Sutton and Smith 1995; Wilson-Barnett et al. 2000). In order to be able to carry out advanced practice activities, an individual needs a particular set of personal characteristics. Much of the literature on this originates from research carried out in nursing, although the characteristics identified might equally apply to other health professionals at the same level of practice (Eddy 2008). The key personal characteristics of advanced practitioners have been identified following an extensive review of the literature, and it is interesting to note that entrepreneurs/innovators share many of the advanced practitioner characteristics listed in Table 2.1, for example, according to Keane (1989), entrepreneurial characteristics include:

- A desire for more freedom in decision-making
- Goal orientation
- Self-motivation
- Self-confidence
- Optimism about their own ability to use the 'system' in order to change things
- Courage.

However, these commonalities should not surprise us, given that it is the entrepreneurial 'spirit' of advanced practitioners that enables them to identify current problems and bring about practice/service improvement for their

Table 2.1 Personal characteristics of advanced practitioners

1. Knowledgeable
2. Understands the system
3. Visionary
4. Risk taker
5. Good interpersonal abilities
6. Confident and motivated
7. Creative critical thinker
8. Goodness
9. Autonomous

organization. Advanced practitioners' key characteristics (Table 2.1) are now discussed with reference to supporting literature:

1. Knowledgeable

According to Mantzoukas and Watkinson's (2007) review of international literature, advanced practitioners have the ability to use many types of knowledge which can be categorized as both theoretical and experiential. Carper (1978) identified ways of knowing in nursing: empirics (scientific), aesthetics (the art of nursing), ethics (a moral sense), and personal (self-awareness) which are each sources of knowledge that, together, give us 'evidence' on which to base practice. Munhall (1993) suggested that 'unknowing' is another important source of knowledge. Through being acutely conscious of particular deficiencies in their knowledge, advanced practitioners avoid immediate recourse to tradition-based decisions and actions, rather, they are alert and responsive to all clues in the current ambiguous situation, and form judgments and perform actions based on those cues (Galle and Whitcombe 2006; Riley et al. 2008).

These practitioners integrate and use their knowledge appropriately in a specific practice situation through the process of critical reasoning and reflection (see item 7). Benner et al. (1996) argue that interpretation of the clinical situation in light of the practitioner's knowledge base is the mechanism whereby the best decisions possible can be made when situations are complex and when certainty is impossible. Important issues for advanced practitioners, therefore, include:

A. Identifying gaps in their knowledge, through individual critical reflection on their own practice.
B. Taking appropriate action to fill these gaps, through, for example:
   • formal Masters level academic preparation
   • work-based learning activities as part of the organization's continuing professional development programme
   • attendance at relevant conferences
   • reading relevant journal articles/research reports/government and professional organization papers.

2. Understands the system

Heath (1998) discusses the importance of socio-political knowing in addition to Carper's (1978) types of knowing. She suggests that in complex situations many local and national influences are likely to operate, for example, having identified local service deficiencies and the needs of the local community, a particular organization will implement a government guideline in a way designed to bring about the local service improvements that are most needed. So advanced practitioners need not only to be aware of all these factors but also to understand how each might impinge on their decision-making processes and decision outcomes.

Lloyd Jones (2005) argues that role transition into a new level of practice is aided by knowing how the organization operates as a socio-political system. Despite this, Flanagan (1998: 698) suggests that political skills are recognized as 'essential survival skills' only when practitioners become more experienced in their role. Thus lack of political understanding may be a cause of delay in implementing the full range of advanced practitioners' role functions when they first start work at that level.

Since advanced practitioners are tasked with introducing and facilitating change in the form of care/service improvements, they must know how decisions are reached in their organization. By knowing these decision-making processes ('having a sense of the game plan' according to Ball and Cox 2004: 18), they will be better able to manipulate the system to bring about change (Butcher and Clarke 2003; Mackey 2007). When the advanced practitioner presents a case for practice/service change in which the politico-social influences are taken into account, then managers may be more likely to consider such a change.

Given that health and social services not only operate as political systems but also as businesses, in order to carry out their practice improvement functions advanced practitioners must have knowledge and abilities related to business planning and budgeting (Douglas and Normand 2005; Hardy and Snaith 2007; Snaith and Hardy 2007; Douglas 2008; Barker 2009). If not prepared adequately for the business-related functions of their role, they will be unable to carry out their role functions fully (Gould 2008). For example, if practitioners propose change which does not fit in with an organization's current business and strategic plans, it may adversely affect their credibility as a manager/leader and increase resistance to future plans for change which they may propose.

3. Visionary

Being a visionary is a 'future-think' characteristic. It involves not only having a vision of how things *might* be but also what actions should be taken to make this vision a reality (Furlong and Smith 2005). The visionary practitioner must be able to decide which innovations will provide most benefit and how best to bring about the innovation in organizational systems or in work practices.

According to Boyatzis and Akrivou (2006: 634), the individual and group must have a clear vision of a feasible future state, towards which end the will and determination of the individuals can be focused. Without a clearly expressed vision, individuals or teams may fall back on re-creating the past, that is, they may rely on traditional ways of doing things in order to continue to 'utilize their strengths and not experiment with new behaviour'. So important is this attribute, that the Foresight Healthcare Panel (2000) stated that the performance of those in positions of responsibility should be evaluated in terms of their ability not only to stimulate but also to sustain innovation (Recommendation 9).

4. Risk taker

Visionary and entrepreneurial practitioners must be not only willing to take risky decisions but also be adept at taking risky decisions. This involves being aware of the uncertainties associated with the process of change and its outcomes (Thompson 1999; Littunen 2000). They must be comfortable with the ambiguities associated with their own decisions and must recognize the importance of balancing potential positive and negative outcomes of risky decisions when seeking to improve practice or services. Their decision-making must be based on a broad range of knowledge so that they can be flexible and improvisational when finding ways around unexpected undesirable outcomes, and in order to capitalize on unexpected desirable outcomes (Leybourne 2006). However, in order to minimize the occurrence of unwanted outcomes, advanced practitioners must operate within their organization's governance and risk management regulations and procedures, which provide a framework by which risk can be judged, related to potential outcomes (NHS Scotland 2007).

5. Interpersonal abilities

In order to operate, Whole Systems must have open channels of communication so that all stakeholders can collaborate freely to bring about integrated care of ever higher quality. Not only are communication and collaborative abilities the key to Whole Systems working but they are also essential characteristics of the advanced practitioner (Hamric et al. 2005).

Interpersonal expertise enables practitioners to network and share their visionary ideas (Por 2008). By developing relationships with other professionals in these interprofessional/stakeholder networks, the practitioner can minimize resistance to innovation and so facilitate change (Ball and Cox 2004). Advanced practitioners generally interact with many other members of the inter-disciplinary team when carrying out their change functions. Because of the uncertainties associated with change in complex organizations, conflict is likely to occur. Therefore, the abilities required to deal with conflicts sensitively and to take preventative action where possible are key applications of interpersonal abilities (Ball and Cox 2004). Service improvement innovations often require use of resources, thus the ability to negotiate for scarce resources is also an essential advanced practitioner characteristic (Manley et al. 2008). Improvements may also require the advanced practitioner to apply their interpersonal abilities when coaching/guiding other staff to develop their knowledge/skills (Hamric et al. 2005). Thus it is through application of their interpersonal expertise that advanced practitioners can enact their role functions and achieve their work-related goals.

6. Confident and motivated

In their meta-analysis of the literature, Judge and Bono (2001) found that self-esteem (the overall value that the individual places on his/her own personal characteristics) and self-efficacy (the individual's estimate of his/her ability to perform successfully in a particular situation) were influential positive indicators of job performance. Self-confidence and mastery (job performance expertise) grow from an individual's experience of repeatedly performing well. Bandura (1989a) argued that people need strong self-efficacy beliefs, as their high expectations of themselves may lead them to seek to achieve them, whereas practitioners with low expectations of themselves would not attempt the challenging tasks that form the core of advanced practice.

Thus in order to be successful, advanced practitioners, who deal with uncertainty, complexity and challenges as part of their roles, should have strong belief in their ability to succeed. As we have seen, this is also a feature of the entrepreneurial character. Self-efficacy can be developed through putting oneself in difficult situations repeatedly and persisting despite all the setbacks that will arise. Through reflecting on their performance, and changing their actions appropriately next time a similar situation arises, gradually individuals build a stronger belief in their abilities, and decision-making is improved (Bandura 1989b).

Confidence in their own ability to apply knowledge appropriately in their decision-making also enables practitioners to gain the respect of colleagues (Lloyd Jones 2005), and lends credibility to the individual practitioner. This has the effect of reducing resistance to any change in practice or service that they are trying to introduce, according to Ball and Cox (2004). Given the complexity of health and social care organizations, success in bringing about change requires persistence in the face of difficulties, and persistence and effort are a consequence of an individual's self-efficacy belief (Bandura and Cervone 1983). As a result, practitioners with high self-efficacy beliefs will make stronger efforts to achieve the task and will persist with their efforts for longer than a person with lower self-efficacy beliefs. Thus practitioners' self-efficacy beliefs influence their motivation.

Staff self-efficacy beliefs and their motivation levels can be adversely affected by an organizational ethos and structure which does not actively encourage entrepreneurial thinking or change. Advanced practitioners must therefore seek to help their organization adopt structures and practices that more closely approach the cultural characteristics associated with an entrepreneurial organization, referred to earlier in this chapter, since such a culture is essential for building and maintaining the efficacy beliefs and motivation of its staff (Thompson 1999).

7. Creative critical thinking

There are different models of creativity, and consequently different research approaches to the study of the concept. From a systems perspective, creative people have been found to be self-motivating, in other words they are creative because they love their work. From a developmental perspective, researchers have suggested that 'creative breakthroughs are possible only after prolonged preparation' (Petrowski 2000: 310). Thus advanced practitioners must spend many years mastering their discipline before achieving the insight which is necessary for creativity to express itself.

Such persistence requires a high level of motivation, which is driven not only by self-efficacy beliefs (see item 6), but also, according to Boyatzis and Akrivou (2006), by an individual's concept of her/his 'ideal self'. Our concept of our 'ideal' is made up of all the elements of 'self' we want to develop. Having such a sense of future-self motivates us to change. Boyatzis and Akrivou (2006: 625) also suggest that our 'ideal-self' 'monitors and guides all actions and decisions in a direction which ensures deeper self-satisfaction'. This sense of self-satisfaction consequently indirectly affects individuals' creative ability, by influencing their motivation.

The skills of metacritiquing or meta-knowing involve thinking about what we're thinking and how we came to think it (Kuhn 1999). When we exercise our metacritiquing abilities, we don't take our own thinking and decisions or those of others on trust, because we accept that thinking and resultant decisions might be flawed. Thus our thinking – the process and product – must be subjected to a frequent critical review as part of critical reflection. This critical review process is essential to development of advanced practitioners' know-that (theoretical) and know-how (experiential) knowledge and to consequent improvement in clinical decision-making and demonstration of competence in evidence-based practice (Mantzoukas and Watkinson 2008).

Experience alone does not guarantee the development of advanced level expertise (Bobay 2004). It is the persistent carrying out of active reflection for many years using critical thinking and metacritiquing skills that may eventually enable creativity to develop. Creative thinking is a useful ability for advanced practitioners to develop, because it is associated with entrepreneurial thinking which involves the challenging of conventional ideas or traditional ways of doing things (McFadzean 1999). Thus creative thinking enables the practitioner to discover new ways of working to overcome problems in patient care and to identify how best to bring about service improvements (Schmid 2004). Creative thinking is discussed further, regarding application of whole systems theory in the management and delivery of healthcare, in Chapter 3.

8. Goodness

All healthcare professionals are in the business of 'caring' and Benner et al. (1996) identified the practitioner's notion of 'goodness' as a key concept underlying caring practice. According to these authors, nurses have a 'disposition towards what is good and right' (1996: 15). This disposition is not only an individual moral sense, but is one that is expressed in the Codes of Conduct which guide the practice all health professionals. As a consequence, practitioners strive to be good because of their strong moral sense of 'goodness' and they also want to do good, that is carry out practice which conforms to this. Because advanced practitioners care about the quality of their own and their team's practice, they are committed to improving it where possible. Good, caring practice demands commitment. Roach (1985: 173) defines commitment as a 'complex affective response characterized by a convergence between one's desires and one's obligations, and by a deliberate choice to act in accordance with them'. Commitment is needed because enacting improvement changes can be a prolonged, difficult process, involving conflict with others in the team or organization and times of self-doubt. Thus 'good' advanced practitioners must have courage as well as a strong self-efficacy belief in order to support their ethical decision-making. Although there is no single template for 'good' ethical decisions, advanced practitioners can build a holistic picture of what 'good' ethical decisions look like, through critical reflection on the personal and professional values which underlie the decisions they have taken (Mackey 2007).

9. Autonomy

Keenan (1999: 561) defines autonomy as 'the exercise of considered, independent judgement to effect a desirable outcome', and many authors identify autonomy as one of the descriptors of advanced practice (Bousfield 1997; Bamford and Gibson 2000; Castledine 2002; Brown and Draye 2003). Indeed, it is so central to advanced practice that, if autonomy is restricted, frustration and consequent de-motivation can result, all of which reduces the ability of individuals to carry out their role functions effectively (Gould 2008). The autonomy associated with advanced practice arises from the practitioner's 'ability to critically and analytically look into experiences, to develop and utilize the multiple types of knowledge and to implement this developed knowledge into practice' (Mantzoukas and Watkinson 2007: 31). According to these authors, such autonomy produces high quality patient care and the development of associated healthcare services.

Keenan (1999) states that in order to act autonomously as an advanced practitioner, the individual must have an appropriate level and scope of knowledge gained through education and experience. Reed and Lawrence (2008) add that having sufficient knowledge now does not give the practitioner the right to take autonomous decisions at some time in the future. The 'right' of advanced practitioners to be autonomous decision-makers is only preserved if they consistently maintain their knowledge base through critical reflection and continuing professional development activities (Carnwell and Daly 2003).

It might be assumed that the goals of interprofessional team working within 'whole systems' could conflict with individual and professional autonomy. However, according to the results of Brown and Draye's (2003) study, individual professional autonomy is essential if practitioners are to be able to demonstrate their ability to their colleagues in the interprofessional team. If practice autonomy is restricted, then a professional's credibility is weakened (see item 6). Similarly, Rafferty et al.'s (2001) study investigating the relationship between interdisciplinary teamwork and nurse autonomy found consistently positive associations. Nurses rating high on teamwork scores also rated highly on autonomy and both were positively correlated with perceptions of improvements in care delivery. Autonomous nurses were also more involved in interprofessional team decision-making. These results suggest that professionals' autonomy should be valued and encouraged.

Case study: Applying personal characteristics (1–9) as an advanced practitioner

Jake is an emergency nurse practitioner who liaised with the motorway police when they were involved in managing and investigating road traffic accidents and/or notifying victims' families. In talking with them, Jake discovered the police were usually first on the scene of major accidents and they expressed interest in knowing how to help victims while waiting for an ambulance to arrive. They agreed it would be mutually beneficial to arrange for Jake to accompany them on patrol, review the range of injuries they commonly witness, assess their training needs in first aid, and advise on the type of equipment they might carry to help stabilize injuries in the short term. On one such occasion they attended a motorcycle accident where the victim (Michelle) was found lying unconscious on a motorway after being thrown off her bike (mechanical failure) into the path of an oncoming vehicle which ran over her leg. Jake supported Michelle's leg with a splint until an ambulance arrived. The severity of the injury meant amputation was probable but, after extensive orthopaedic and plastic surgery, Michelle's leg was saved. This outcome would have been unlikely without Jake's early immobilization of the leg (it was flapping about in the draught of passing traffic).

Jake applied all nine characteristics associated with an advanced practitioner. While these largely correspond with matrix model themes and registered nurses

(Chapter 1), 'visionary' and 'risk taker' qualities distinguish the advanced practitioner. Jake was visionary in understanding how his expertise was transferable beyond the A&E department, where he normally worked, to enhance the role of the motorway police who, in turn, were better equipped to give first aid to victims in the precious moments before an ambulance came. He was a risk taker, both in terms of being innovative, and in exposing himself to physical danger while administering first aid on a motorway.

Summary of the personal characteristics of advanced practitioners

In this section of the chapter, the mix of personal attributes required of advanced practitioners has been discussed in relation to their potential effects on advanced practice and decision-making. However, each characteristic does not function independently, rather they have a synergistic effect, and together they act as prerequisites for the decision-making expertise demanded of an effective advanced practitioner. The case study (real event – identities changed to maintain anonymity) illustrated how all nine characteristics combine, with a particular emphasis upon visionary and risk taker qualities of advanced practitioners.

Reflective activity 2.1

Aim: to help you fit more comfortably into your advanced practice role, by helping you identify targets for development of your personal characteristics.

In relation to the personal characteristics discussed in this chapter, carry out this reflective exercise, writing down your conclusions. Try to answer the following questions as honestly as possible.

- Which of the characteristics, listed in Table 2.1 do you have?
- What would your 'ideal self' be like?
- Which abilities do you need to develop further in order to approach your 'ideal self'?

Following this individual reflection on your own personal characteristics, ask one or more work friends/colleagues to do the following:

- Read the characteristics you've identified and
- Discuss with you their own view about your attributes and those that have scope for further development.

In light of your own and your colleagues' reflections:

- Identify three characteristics you'd like to improve, then
- Decide on specific actions you can take to improve these characteristics.

Advanced practice: conceptual confusion

There is no internationally/nationally agreed definition of advanced professional practice as various authors have pointed out (Pearson and Peels 2002; Bryant-Lukosius et al. 2004; Fawcett and Graham 2005; Gardner et al. 2007; Eddy 2008). As a result of the diverse definitions of advanced practice, a profusion of associated role titles has developed. Examples related to nursing include: nurse practitioner, advanced nurse practitioner, clinical nurse specialist, advanced clinical nurse specialist, advanced practice nurse. The necessary knowledge and skills associated with these roles are not standardized which has made it impossible for other professionals, patients and managers to know which levels of autonomy and accountability are associated with these roles; consequently considerable confusion has arisen about what an individual in a particular role can or should do (Furlong and Smith 2005).

An agreed national definition is essential as it forms the basis for determining the standards which are appropriate to an advanced level of practice. These standards, in turn, will act as a framework on which the quality and efficiency outcomes of an advanced practice role can be identified and evaluated. In recognition of the importance of arriving at a common definition, the government is working with the various health professions' regulatory bodies to achieve this end (DH 2008a).

However, the basic meaning of advanced practice is practice at a level beyond that of initial professional registration, with its associated increase in knowledge and skills. According to some authors, advanced practice is viewed as primarily direct, 'hands-on' patient care (Donnelly 2006). However, in addition to direct forms of practice, Aranda and Jones (2008) identify more distal forms of advanced practice involving the practitioner in manipulation of the field of advanced practice in which, for example, coordination of care or leadership or improving the practice of others are equally important aspects of the role.

If field-of-practice functions as well as direct-care functions are both recognized as elements of advanced practice, then professionals who are not mainly (or at all) directly involved in patient care can be considered advanced practitioners. However, there is a danger inherent in 'distal' practice: that it may be viewed as a solely management function, and practitioners may lose their focus on patients (Aranda and Jones 2008). It is, therefore, the individual responsibility of practitioners in such roles to maintain a patient-focus in their decision-making.

Different levels of practice

The Department of Health recognized that there are differing levels of practice beyond initial registration. As a result a first career framework for nurses, midwives and health visitors was produced (DH 1999: 32–5), in which two 'ranges' of practice beyond initial registration were identified: those of senior registered practitioner and consultant.

In this early vision of career progression, senior practitioners were viewed as clinicians who had:

- significant clinical/public health leadership and/or
- clinical management and/or
- specialist care functions.

The role functions of such a practitioner were similar to those of (the then) current senior clinicians or managers. However, the novel element in this description is the leadership function. In this document (DH 1999: 33–5), the government made it clear that any changes it proposed were aimed at strengthening professional leadership primarily in order to bring about improvement of patient services. At this level of practice, leadership was not envisaged as a necessary function, although it was expected that some roles might demand a leadership component.

A new level, that of consultant practice, was designed specifically to lead change aimed at improving quality and services. Consultants' areas of responsibility were identified as:

- Expert practice;
- Professional leadership and consultancy;
- Education and development;
- Practice and service development linked to research and evaluation (DH 1999: 33).

It was recognized that consultants may or may not have a specialist level of qualification, and that it is a practitioner's level of role responsibilities and competences which determine whether or not an individual is functioning at a consultant level.

Career ladder

Since the government's initial work on career development for nurses, midwives and health visitors, they have identified, along with healthcare professional regulatory bodies, the need to create a coherent career framework, in which levels of practice are identified for all types of health workers (Secretary of State for Health 2007). This work is being carried out by the Skills for Health Organization, which is a UK-wide independent organization, funded by the UK Health Departments, the Sector Skills Development Agency, education regulatory bodies as well as Health Sector Employers and Providers (www.concordat.org.uk/signatories/fullsignatories/skillsforhealth. cfm). Working with its partners, it has identified a career ladder applicable to all health professionals and support staff which recognizes stepped levels of competence-based practice (Table 2.2) www.skillsforhealth.org.uk/page/ career-frameworks). The number of post-registration levels of practice has

Table 2.2 Career framework for health

Level	Description of level
9	More senior staff
8	Consultant practitioners
7	Advanced practitioners
6	Senior practitioners/specialist practitioners
5	Practitioners
4	Assistant practitioners/associate practitioners
3	Senior healthcare assistants/technicians
2	Support workers
I	Initial entry level jobs

www.skillsforhealth.org.uk/page/career-frameworks/ (accessed 28 July 2008)

been increased from two to four, in recognition of the ever expanding scope of practice of health professionals.

Competences

The Knowledge and Skills Framework set out the competences associated with the levels of practice identified in the *Agenda for Change* document (DH 2004). However, these competences only apply to staff in the NHS. The Skills for Health Organization has been tasked with identifying competences for all staff in health-related occupations in any organization, not just the NHS, in line with the government's demand for integrated service delivery. They define a competence as a description of 'what individuals need to do and know in order to carry out specific work activities. It sets out the performance criteria to be met and the knowledge and understanding required to undertake the activities successfully' (DH 2008b:9).

The value of identifying competences which are skills- and knowledge-based is that a practitioner/manager can:

- Identify the mix that best suits local practice and service development needs
- Identify which mix of competencies a practitioner has and from this decide the level at which the practitioner is working
- Guide individuals to develop competences to the appropriate level, where lacking currently, in order to fit in with local service needs and to progress their own career.

The Skills for Health Organization has identified four different types of competences (Table 2.3). In a fast changing health service, the traditional, single form of career progression that is vertical will become less common, as more 'managing' and 'leading' functions become the remit of all professionals. In

Table 2.3 Types of competence

- **Generic** – apply equally across all UK work sectors (not just the health sector), e.g. competences describing management or learning and development functions
- **Common** – apply to all healthcare roles, and to some social care roles, but not to other sectors, e.g. competencies describing interactions and relationships with patients/clients
- **Shared** – applying to a sub-set of roles/practitioners in some contexts only, e.g. those relating to the planning and provision of treatment and care
- **Specific** – to a given context, setting or patient group and not relevant beyond that, e.g. those relating to perioperative or neonatal care.

www.skillsforhealth.org.uk/page/career-frameworks/allied-health-professions (accessed 28 July 2008)

this environment, individuals with an identified mix of transferable (generic, common, shared) competences will then have the career options of moving either:

- vertically to the next level up, or
- sideways to a new job that matches most of their particular competence-mix.

(Veres and Sims 1999)

Both pathways will be facilitated by selection of an appropriate mix of further experience, formal education and continuing professional development activities. Sideways career movement affords increased flexibility to healthcare managers in their workforce planning and service development activities, as well as to individual practitioners when planning their career progression (DH 2007; 2008a; 2008c).

Work on identifying the key competences that an individual health worker needs in order to practise at each of the nine levels is ongoing. However, even when competences have been mapped for each level and role in each profession, it is recognized that competences will need to be re-configured at intervals, as professions and services continually develop through time. It is also recognized that practitioners in one particular role may have a different mix of competences because role competences address the specific needs of the local organization and particular patient groups. Up-to-date information on the competences identified for different professional groups (e.g. allied health professionals and public health professionals), levels of practice and roles can be accessed via the Skills for Health Organization's website (www.skillsforhealth.org.uk).

Prior to the current work of the Skills for Health Organization, individual professional regulatory bodies and/or colleges had, to a greater or lesser extent, identified the characteristics of their own profession's advanced practice and associated competences. However, the Skills for Health Organization's careers framework will increasingly become the 'common currency', and all healthcare professions' regulatory bodies are in the process of agreeing how their current various 'Senior practitioner', 'Advanced' and 'Consultant' definitions and roles fit into the career framework categories and agreeing on common/shared transferable competencies (DH 2008a: 40).

At the same time, the Council for Healthcare Regulatory Excellence (CHRE) is seeking to integrate the work of Professional Regulatory bodies and the Skills for Health Organization with European and international standards (www.nmc-uk.org/). This process should produce an internationally recognized framework of levels of competence in heath-related jobs and so help reduce the confusion which has hitherto existed.

Senior/specialist, advanced and consultant practitioners

Working with all its partners, the Skills for Health Organization has provided an overview of senior/specialist, advanced and consultant practitioners' levels of practice (Table 2.4) (www.skillsforhealth.org.uk/page/career-frameworks). These outlines are deliberately broad in scope, so that they are relevant to all health professions.

Table 2.4 Career framework for health (extract)

Level	Description of level
8.	**Consultant practitioners** Staff working at a very high level of clinical expertise and/or have responsibility for planning of services.
7.	**Advanced practitioners** Experienced clinical professionals who have developed their skills and theoretical knowledge to a very high standard. They are empowered to make high-level clinical decisions and will often have their own caseload. Non-clinical staff at level 7 will typically be managing a number of service areas.
6.	**Senior practitioners/specialist practitioners** Staff who would have a higher degree of autonomy and responsibility than 'practitioners' in the clinical environment, or who would be managing one or more service areas in the non-clinical environment.

www.skillsforhealth.org.uk/page/career-frameworks/ (accessed 28 July 2008)

The difference between these levels of practice relate to the depth and scope of knowledge and expertise of individual practitioners. Those involved in taking strategic decisions (level 8), have a broader and deeper knowledge of the Whole Systems working of their organization than either level 6 or 7 practitioners. Level 6 practitioners have responsibilities focused on direct, clinical practice and management activities related to a specific patient group or service.

The advanced level of practice (level 7)

Descriptors have been identified which outline, under eight headings, the categories of responsibilities of each level of practitioners, and those which relate to level 7 are identified in Appendix 2.1. These descriptors have been structured so that they are relevant to all health practitioner disciplines (e.g. occupational therapists, radiographers) and roles (e.g. advanced neonatal nurse, advanced podiatrist).

Traditionally advanced practitioners were perceived as mainly clinical practitioners who delivered direct care, as discussed previously. However, it has since been recognized that many carry out non-clinical functions (Por 2008). As a result, the descriptors identify the inter-linked educative, management and leadership, research and clinical elements which make up the advanced practitioner level of practice. Generally, the advanced practitioner's work is not limited to just one of these elements, but involves a mix of them. Such a mix results in a composite set of descriptors and associated competences which identify the requirements of a specific role.

Since these descriptors apply to all health workers, they are sometimes complex and multi-faceted, and, as a result, they must be read carefully so that the particular elements of each descriptor which apply to individual practitioners can be identified. Given the difficulty involved in fully incorporating all health work at each level, descriptors are being modified in an ongoing process. Appendix 2.1 illustrates the descriptors as modified in January 2008, but for further updates the reader is advised to access the Skills for Health Organization's website. Key issues associated with the descriptors outlined in Appendix 1 are now discussed with reference to supporting literature.

Scope of independent decision-making

As can be seen in Descriptor 5 (Appendix 2.1), advanced practitioners are *accountable* for direct care and quality improvement decisions related to their own patient group/case load. However, they are only *responsible* for a whole work area/clinical pathway, since the accountability and final decision-making rest with a higher level practitioner or management team. Nevertheless, being 'responsible' requires advanced practitioners to exercise their judgment expertise in order to provide decision-makers with evidence on which to base their decisions. As a consequence, advanced practitioners should form part of the team concerned with managing their specialist service/care pathway/work area. Thus, for example, a consultant who leads a particular service will be aware of the organization's strategic plans as well as developments occurring in services which impinge on her/his own. S/he will take the advice of advanced practitioners, who have expertise in direct care and management functions within the service, in order to formulate and initiate improvements in the service. Since these improvements will be based on evidence from advanced practitioners and the consultant's own knowledge of the system, they will mesh with other current and planned organizational changes and will promote effective Whole Systems working (DH 2005).

Expert practice

Underpinning the descriptors in Appendix 2.1 is the notion of expertise. According to Benner (1984), development to an expert level of practice requires at least five years' experience at post-registration level and assumes that the practitioner has been working in the same clinical environment for that amount of time. McSherry and Johnson (2005) suggest a longer in-practice time is needed as preparation for consultant level posts (a minimum of ten years). However, the current expertise demonstrated by an advanced practitioner is not by itself sufficient to designate an individual as an 'advanced' level practitioner. Rather, the critical features of advanced practice expertise are that it must be:

- Demonstrable, in terms of current competences
- Seen to be expanding, through the individual's development of further competences
- Utilized to improve practice or services, as discussed earlier in this chapter.

Leadership

The government states that increasing the leadership potential of professionals is central to their vision for improving healthcare outcomes, and that all practitioners in advanced level roles must be leaders of practice or service development (DH 2008a). This requirement is recognized overtly in Descriptor 2 (Appendix 2.1), but is also implicit within the others (Descriptors 1–8). Leadership in advanced practice roles is concerned with the promotion and development of clinical practice directly and through policy implementation. Whereas, according to Hardy and Snaith (2007), at consultant level, leadership is mainly concerned with developing clinical practice and services through decision-making about the organization's strategic direction, and associated policy development and evaluation strategies.

There are several perspectives on leadership in the literature (Kark et al. 2003; Padilla et al. 2007; Snaith and Hardy 2007). However the notion of transformational leadership has been used by the NHS Institute for Innovation and Improvement to identify the qualities required by NHS leaders (www.nhsleadershipqualities.nhs.uk). Through their personal characteristics, credibility and actions, transformational leaders gain for themselves and for others in the team 'a voice in the development of services [and] a sense of ownership and influence' (Hurley and Linsley 2007: 753). Primarily, they seek organizational power in order to use it to empower their followers or others in the team to achieve organizational goals, not for personal reasons such as career progression (Guest et al. 2004; Yun et al. 2006). This moral basis of transformational leadership is noted by several authors (Kark et al. 2003; Gardner et al. 2005; Mackey 2007; Padilla et al. 2007).

Although they must lead when appropriate, in the integrated team-work central to effective Whole Systems working, advanced practitioners will not take the leader role on every occasion. In some situations or projects, the particular competence mix of other team members will make them more appropriate leaders. So advanced practitioners must also be expert at working cooperatively towards team goals under the leadership of another professional (Fitzgerald 2006; Callaghan 2008).

Educator

Advanced practitioners are required to help others in the team recognize their knowledge gaps and associated practice limitations. This might be achieved through coaching/mentoring individuals, or by leading group reflection sessions set up to critically evaluate the team's activities and outcomes (Lockyer et al. 2004). In these sessions, relationships between practice outcomes, their precursor decisions and knowledge base can each be identified and gaps recognized. Then the advanced practitioner can decide upon appropriate training and development activities which would appropriately address these gaps (Appendix 2.1, Descriptor 7).

Researcher/service developer

According to the literature, producing knowledge for the profession and health service by undertaking research is the descriptor (Appendix 2.1, Descriptor 8) least displayed by advanced practitioners (Guest et al. 2004). There seems to be a reliance on others to carry out research, the relevant findings of which these practitioners apply in their organization's activities. However, even when research-derived knowledge is available, there is considerable time lag between knowledge production and knowledge implementation in practice (Sherriff et al. 2007). The advanced practitioner therefore has a major function in 'evidence-brokering' (Gerrish et al. 2007), and developing evidenced-based practice, by:

- disseminating relevant research results,
- helping the team to implement research findings and
- involving the team in research related to their local practice and services.

Given the budgetary constraints of healthcare organizations, unless advanced practitioners can demonstrate that improvements stem from their work, they may be perceived as an expensive and unnecessary addition to the staffing budget and their roles will disappear. Therefore advanced practitioners must be regularly involved in planning and carrying out evaluation of their role outcomes (Middleton et al. 2007).

Reflective activity 2.2

Critically reflect on two recent work situations, one which made you feel dissatisfied and one in which you were satisfied with your performance. Then carry out this exercise, identifying, in as much detail as you can, the good/improvable factors.

In relation to the practice elements discussed in this chapter:

* Identify the elements of your own practice which you think you have developed most fully.
* Identify those elements which you believe need further development.
* Work out strategies by which you might develop those aspects of your role with which you are currently dissatisfied.

Summary

Emphasis on competences alone is not sufficient to describe advanced practitioners or their practice. It is the blend of their personal characteristics (discussed in the first section of this chapter) which allows practitioners to continuously develop their competences. Thus it is the combination of practice competences and personal characteristics that, together, explain what advanced practitioners can do and how they are able to do it (Mantzoukas and Watkinson 2007).

Advanced practitioners gain satisfaction from the challenge of taking complex decisions in new and ambiguous situations that may involve consideration of multiple interacting factors. The entrepreneurial functions which these practitioners carry out for their employers (categorized as Descriptors 9 in Appendix 1), result from application of their complex decision-making abilities. Advanced practitioners therefore make a positive contribution to their employing organization, by:

* constantly moving their organization forward
* meeting government policy demands
* providing health services of ever higher quality.

Based on this chapter's review of the literature related to advanced practitioners and their practice, it might be argued that the decision-making expertise of advanced practitioners is an important factor contributing to the continuing success of their organization.

Key points

* Advanced practitioners are experienced health professionals with advanced knowledge and skills, empowered to take complex clinical decisions and manage caseloads/areas of practice.

- Personal characteristics associated with advanced practitioners' include: understands system, visionary, risk taker, confident/motivated, creative critical thinker, goodness, and autonomous.
- Advanced practitioners share similarities with entrepreneurs and innovators in accepting the challenge of continually developing systems and practices to meet current and future demands.
- Skills for Health Organization's descriptors of advanced practice identify: specialized knowledge, supervision, managing change, specialist practice, managerial, educational, and research competences.
- Advanced practitioners are collaborative leaders who mentor/supervise/empower others to promote high standards of care, achieve organizational goals, and transform clinical practice.
- Effective advanced practice is achieved where advanced practitioner personal characteristics are successfully blended with the competences identified by the Skills for Health Organization.

References

Aranda, K. and Jones, A. (2008) Exploring new advanced practice roles in community nursing: a critique. *Nursing Inquiry*, 15(1): 3–10.

Ball, C. and Cox, C.I. (2004) Part two: The core components of legitimate influence and the conditions that constrain or facilitate advanced nursing practice in adult critical care. *International Journal of Nursing Practice*, 10: 10–20.

Bamford, O. and Gibson, F. (2000) The clinical nurse specialist: perceptions of practicing CNSs of their role and development needs. *Journal of Clinical Nursing*, 9: 282–92.

Bandura, A. (1989a) Perceived self efficacy in the exercise of personal agency. *The Psychologist*, 2: 411–24.

Bandura, A. (1989b) Human agency in social cognitive theory. *American Psychologist*, 44(9): 1175–84.

Bandura, A. and Cervone, D. (1983) Self evaluative and self-efficacy mechanisms governing the motivational effects of goal systems. *Journal of Personality and Psychology*, 45: 1017–28.

Barker, A.M. (ed.) (2009) *Advanced Practice Nursing: Essential knowledge for the profession.* Sudbury, MA: Jones and Bartlett.

Benner, P. (1984) *From Novice to Expert: Excellence and power in clinical nursing practice.* Menlo Park, CA: Addison-Wesley.

Benner, P., Tanner, C.A. and Chesla, C.A. (1996) *Expertise in Nursing Practice: Caring, clinical judgment and ethics.* New York: Springer.

Bobay, K.L.F. (2004) Does experience really matter? *Nursing Science Quarterly*, 17(4): 313–16.

Bousfield, C. (1997) A phenomenological investigation into the role of the clinical nurse specialist. *Journal of Advanced Nursing*, 25: 245–56.

Boyatzis, R.E. and Akrivou, K. (2006) The ideal self as the driver of intentional change. *Journal of Management Development*, 25(7): 624–42.

Brown, M.A. and Draye, M.A. (2003) Experiences of pioneer nurse practitioners in establishing advanced practice roles. *Journal of Nursing Scholarship*, 4th Quarter: 391–7.

Bryant-Lukosius, D., DiCensio, A., Browne, G. and Pinelli, J. (2004) Advanced practice nursing roles: development, implementation and evaluation. *Journal of Advanced Nursing,* 48(5): 519–29.

Butcher, D. and Clarke, M. (2003) Redefining managerial work: smart politics. *Management Decision,* 41(5): 477–87.

Callaghan, L. (2008) Advanced nursing practice: an idea whose time has come. *Journal of Clinical Nursing,* 17: 205–13.

Carnwell, R. and Daly, W.M. (2003) Advanced nursing practitioners in primary care settings: an exploration of the developing roles. *Journal of Clinical Nursing,* 12: 630–42.

Carper, B.A. (1978) Fundamental patterns of knowing in nursing. *Advances in Nursing Science,* 1(1): 13–23.

Castledine, G. (2002) Higher level practice is in fact advanced practice. *British Journal of Nursing,* 11: 1166–67.

Department of Health (DH) (1997) *The New NHS: Modern and dependable.* London: TSO.

Department of Health (DH) (1999) *Making a Difference: Strengthening the nursing, midwifery and health visiting contribution to health and healthcare.* London: DH.

Department of Health (DH) (2004) *Agenda for Change, Final Agreement.* www.dh.gov.uk/ Publicationsandstatistics/Publications/PublicationsPolicyAndGuidance/ DH_4095943 (accessed 15 January 2007).

Department of health (DH) (2005) *Improvement Leaders' Guide. Working in systems: Process and systems thinking.* www.dh.gov.uk/en/Publicationsandstatistics/ Publications/PublicationsPolicyAndGuidance/DH_4010092 (accessed 20 January 2009).

Department of Health (DH) (2007*) Towards a Framework for Post Registration Nursing Careers – Consultation Document.* www.dh.gov.uk/en/Consultations/ Liveconsultations/DH_079911 (accessed 12 June 2008).

Department of Health (DH) (2008a) *A High Quality Workforce: NHS next stage review.* London: DH.

Department of Health (DH) (2008b) *Modernising Allied Health Professions (AHP) Careers: A competence-based career framework.* www.dh.gov.uk/en/publicationsandstatistics/ Publications/PublicationsPolicyAndGuidance/DH_086264 (accessed 20 December 2008).

Department of Health (DH) (2008c) *Towards a Framework for Post-registration Nursing Careers: Consultation response report.* www.dh.gov.uk/en/Consultations/ Responsestoconsultations/DH_086465 (accessed 10 August 2008).

Donnelly, G. (2006) The essence of advanced nursing practice. *The Internet Journal of Advanced Nursing Practice,* 8(1).

Douglas, M. (2008) Management roles in nursing: current issues, perspectives and responses (Editorial). *Journal of Nursing Management,* 16: 765–7.

Douglas, H-R. and Normand, C. (2005) Economic evaluation: what does a nurse manager need to know? *Journal of Nursing Management,* 13(5): 419–27.

Eddy, A. (2008) Advanced practice for therapy radiographers – A discussion paper. *Radiography,* 14: 24–31.

Fawcett, J. and Graham, I. (2005) Advanced practice nursing: continuation of the dialogue. *Nursing Science Quarterly,* 18: 37–41.

Fitzgerald, L. (2006) *Managing Change and Role Enactment in the Professionalised Organisation.* Report to the National Coordinating Centre for NHS Service Delivery and Organisation. February. www.sdo.nihr.ac.uk/files/project/21-final-report.pdf (accessed 13th February 2007).

Flanagan, M. (1998) Factors influencing tissue viability nurse specialities in the UK. *British Journal of Nursing*, 7: 690–2.

Foresight Healthcare Panel (2000) *Health Care 2020*. Report for the Department of Trade and Industry. London: TSO.

Fuller, T. and Warren, L. (2006) Entrepreneurship as foresight: a complex social network perspective on organizational foresight. *Futures*, 38: 956–1071.

Furlong, E. and Smith, R. (2005) Advanced nursing practice: policy, education and role development. *Journal of Clinical Nursing*, 14: 1059–66.

Galle, L. and Whitcombe, S.W. (2006) An exploration of ways of knowing employed within occupational therapy. *British Journal of Occupational Therapy*, 69(4): 187–91.

Gardner, G., Chang, A. and Duffield, C. (2007) Making nursing work: breaking through the role confusion of advanced practice nursing. *Journal of Advanced Nursing*, 57(4): 382–91.

Gardner, W.L., Avolio, B.J., Luthans, F., May, D.R. and Walumbwa, F. (2005) 'Can you see the real me?' A self-based model of authentic leader and follower development. *The Leadership Quarterly*, 16: 343–72.

Gerrish, K. Guillaume, L. Kirshbaum et al. (2007) *Empowering Frontline Staff to Deliver Evidence-based Care: The contribution of nurses in advanced practice roles*. Research Report Executive Summary. October. Sheffield Hallam University.

Gould, D. (2008) The matron's role in acute National Health Service Trusts. *Journal of Nursing Management*, 16: 804–12.

Guest, D.E., Pecci, R., Rosenthal, P. et al. (2004) *An Evaluation of the Impact of Nurse, Midwife and Health Visitor Consultants*. Research Report for National Nursing Research Unit. September. www.kcl.ac.uk/school/nursing/nnru/ (accessed 30 October 2007).

Hamric, A. Spross, J. and Hanson, C. (2005) *Advanced Practice Nursing*, 3rd edn. St Louis, MO: Elsevier Saunders.

Hardy, M. and Snaith, B. (2007) How to achieve consultant practitioner status: A discussion paper. *Radiography*, 13: 265–70.

Heath, H. (1998) Reflection and patterns of knowing in nursing. *Journal of Advanced Nursing*, 27(5): 1054–9.

Hurley, J. and Linsley, P. (2007) Leadership challenges to move nurses towards collaborative individualism within a neo-corporate bureaucratic environment. *Journal of Nursing Management*, 15: 749–55.

Judge, T.A. and Bono, J.E. (2001) Relationship of core self-evaluation traits – self-esteem, generalized self-efficacy, locus of control and emotional stability – with job satisfaction and job performance: a meta-analysis. *Journal of Applied Psychology*, 86(1): 80–92.

Kark, R., Shamir, B. and Chen, G. (2003) The two faces of transformational leadership: empowerment and dependency. *Journal of Applied Psychology*, 88(2): 246–55.

Keane, L. (1989) Independent Nurse Consultants: the lateral leap, in R. Pratt and G. Gray (eds) *Issues in Australian Nursing*, 2nd edn. Edinburgh: Churchill Livingstone.

Keenan, J. (1999) A concept analysis of autonomy. *Journal of Advanced Nursing*, 29(3): 556–62.

Kuhn, D. (1999) A developmental model of critical thinking. *Educational Researcher*, 28(2): 16–26.

Leybourne, S.A. (2006) Managing improvisation within change management: lessons from UK financial services. *The Service Industries Journal*, 26(1): 73–95.

Littunen, H. (2000) Entrepreneurship and the characteristics of the entrepreneurial character. *International Journal of Entrepreneurial Behaviour and Research*, 6(6): 295–309.

Lloyd Jones, M. (2005) Role development and effective practice in specialist and advanced practice roles in acute hospital settings: systematic review and meta-synthesis. *Journal of Advanced Nursing,* 49(2): 191–209.

Lockyer, J. Gondocz, T. and Thivierge, R.L. (2004) Knowledge translation: the role and place of practice reflection. *Journal of Continuing Education in the Health Professions,* 24: 50–6.

Mackey, H. (2007) "Do not ask me to remain the same': Foucault and the professional identities of occupational therapists. *Australian Occupational Therapy Journal,* 54: 95–102.

Manley, K., Webster, J., Hale, N., Hayes, N. and Minardi, H. (2008) Leadership role of consultant nurses working with older people: a co-operative enquiry. *Journal of Nursing Management,* 16: 147–58.

Mantzoukas, S. and Watkinson, S. (2007) Review of advanced nursing practice: the international literature and developing the generic features. *Journal of Clinical Nursing,* 16: 28–37.

Mantzoukas, S. and Watkinson, S. (2008) Redescribing reflective practice and evidence-based practice discourses. *International Journal of Nursing Practice,* 14: 129–34.

McFadzean, E. (1999) Encouraging creative thinking. *Leadership and Organization,* 20(7): 374–83.

McSherry, R. and Johnson, S. (eds) (2005) *Demystifying the Nurse/Therapist Consultant.* Cheltenham: Nelson Thornes.

Middleton, S., Allnutt, J., Griffiths, R., McMaster, R., O'Connell, J. and Hillege, J. (2007) Identifying measures for evaluating new models of nursing care: A survey of NSW nurse practitioners. *International Journal of Nursing Practice,* 13: 331–40.

Munhall, P. (1993) 'Unknowing': towards another pattern of knowing in nursing. *Nursing Outlook,* 41(3): 125–8.

NHS Education for Scotland (NES) (2007) *Advanced Practice Succession Planning Pathway.* www.nes.scot.nhs.uk/nursing/roledevelopment/advanced practice/ (accessed 16 December 2008).

NHS Institute for Innovation and Improvement (2008) *NHS Leadership Qualities Framework.* www.nhsleadershipqualities.nhs.uk/ (accessed 12 August 2008).

NHS Scotland (2007) *Clinical Governance Educational Resources.* www.clinicalgovernance.scot.nhs.uk/ (accessed 13 July 2008).

Padilla, A., Hogan, R. and Kaiser, R.B. (2007) The toxic triangle: destructive leaders, susceptible followers, and conducive environments. *The Leadership Quarterly,* 18: 176–94.

Pearson, A. and Peels, S. (2002) Advanced practice in nursing: international perspective. *International Journal of Nursing Practice,* 8, supplement: S1–S4.

Petrowski, M.J. (2000) Creativity research: implications for teaching, learning and thinking. *Reference Service Review,* 28(4): 304–12.

Por, J. (2008) A critical engagement with the concept of advancing nursing practice. *Journal of Nursing Management,* 16: 84–90.

Rafferty, A.M., Ball, J. and Aiken, L.H. (2001) Are teamwork and professional autonomy compatible, and do they result in improved hospital care? *Quality in Health Care,* 10: 32–6.

Reed, P.G. and Lawrence, L.A. (2008) A paradigm for the production of practice-based knowledge. *Journal of Nursing Management,* 16: 422–32.

Riley, J., Beal, J.A. and Lancaster, D. (2008) Scholarly nursing practice from the perspectives of experienced nurses. *Journal of Advanced Nursing,* 61(4): 425–35.

Roach, S.M. (1985) A foundation for nursing ethics, in A. Carmi and S. Schneider (eds) *Nursing, Law and Ethics.* Berlin: Springer-Verlag.

Schmid, T. (2004) Meanings of creativity within occupational therapy practice. *Australian Occupational Therapy Journal*, 51: 80–8.

Secretary of State for Health (2007) *Trust, Assurance and Safety: The Regulation of Health Professionals in the 21st Century*. White Paper, Cm 7013. February. London: TSO.

Sherriff, K.I., Wallis, M. and Chaboyer, W. (2007) Nurses' attitudes to and perceptions of knowledge and skills regarding evidence-based practice. *International Journal of Nursing Practice*, 13: 363–9.

Skills for Health Organization (2009) *Definition of Levels of Practice*. www.skillsforhealth.org.uk/js/uploaded/uploadedablefile3.pdf (accessed 28 February 2009).

Snaith, B. and Hardy, M. (2007) How to achieve advanced practitioner status: A discussion paper. *Radiography*, 13: 142–6.

Sutton, F. and Smith, C. (1995) Advanced nursing practice: new ideas and new perspectives. *Journal of Advanced Nursing*, 21: 1037–43.

Thompson, J.L. (1999) A strategic perspective of entrepreneurship. *International Journal of Entrepreneurial Behaviour and Research*, 5(6): 279–96.

Veres, J.G. and Sims, R.R. (1999) Keys to employee success: what skills are really important for success in the future?, in R.R. Sims and J.G. Veres (eds) *Keys to Employee Success in Coming Decades*. Westport, CT: Quorum Books.

Wilson-Barnett, J., Barriball, L., Reynolds, H., Jowett, S. and Ryrie, I. (2000) Recognizing advanced nursing practice: evidence from two observational studies. *International Journal of Nursing Studies*, 37: 389–400.

Yun, S., Cox, J. and Sims, H.P. (2006) The forgotten follower: a contingency model of leadership and follower self-leadership. *Journal of Managerial Psychology*, 21(4): 374–88.

APPENDIX 2.1
Framework descriptors for Level 7 (Jan 2008)

1. Knowledge, skills, training and experience

Utilizes highly developed specialized knowledge covering a range of procedures and underpinned by relevant broad-based knowledge, experience and competence

AND uses highly specialized theoretical and practical knowledge, some of which is at the forefront of knowledge in the work area. This knowledge forms the basis for originality in developing and/or applying ideas

AND develops new skills in response to emerging knowledge and techniques.

OR

Demonstrates critical awareness of knowledge issues in the work area and at the interface between different or new work areas, creating a research-based diagnosis to problems by integrating knowledge

AND makes judgements with incomplete or limited information developing new skills in response to emerging knowledge and techniques.

2. Supervision

Demonstrates leadership and innovation in work contexts that are unfamiliar, complex and unpredictable and that require solving problems involving many interacting factors.

OR

Reviews strategic impact/outcomes of the work or team.

3. Professional and Vocational Competence

Demonstrates independence in the direction of practice and a high level of understanding of development processes

AND responds to social/scientific, clinical/ethical issues that are encountered in work or study

AND manages change within a complex environment.

OR

Demonstrates independence in the direction of practice responding to social, scientific, clinical and ethical issues that are encountered in work or study

AND has high level of understanding of development processes.

OR

Demonstrates independence in the direction of practice responding to social, scientific, clinical and ethical issues that are encountered in work or study

AND solves problems by integrating complex knowledge sources that are sometimes incomplete, and in new and unfamiliar contexts.

OR

Demonstrates independence in the direction of practice responding to social, scientific, clinical and ethical issues that are encountered in work or study

AND manages change within a complex environment.

4. Analytical/Clinical Skills and Patient Care

Provides highly specialist clinical, technical and/or scientific services,

AND makes complex judgements

OR

Provides highly specialist clinical, technical and/or scientific services across a work area

AND makes complex judgements

OR

Accountable for direct delivery of part of service

AND makes complex judgements.

5. Organizational Skills and Autonomy/Freedom to Act

Responsible for work area, specialist services or clinical pathways

OR

Accountable for direct delivery of part of a service.

6. Planning, Policy and Service Delivery

Proposes changes to practices or procedures which impact beyond own work area

OR

May plan and/or organize a broad range of complex activities or programmes with formulation of strategies.

7. Financial, Administration, Physical and Human Resources

Devises training or development programmes

OR

Responsible for work area budget

OR

Manages staff and/or services ranging in size and complexity

8. Research and Development

Initiates and develops local R and D programmes

www.skillsforhealth.org.uk/js/uploaded/
CF%20Descriptors%20jan%202008.3.pdf (accessed 28 July 2008)

3 Creative thinking for whole systems working

Carolyn Jackson and Peter Ellis

Overview

This chapter will explore the concept of health and social care organizations as complex adaptive systems that face significant challenges if they are to adapt to whole systems (non-linear) working which can respond creatively to changing government policy and continuous NHS reform. It explores and analyses the importance of developing and applying complexity theory to understand the unpredictability of non-linear whole systems and the importance of creative thinking in managing uncertainty – a prerequisite to working effectively as an advanced practitioner (AP) in constantly changing environments of care. It provides practical ways of relating whole systems working to enhance the AP's everyday practice through the use of reflective activities.

Objectives

- Describe the principles of a whole systems approach to health and social care delivery
- Identify the strengths and limitations of whole systems working
- Distinguish non-linear 'living' from linear 'mechanical' organizational systems
- Identify ways to develop creative thinking skills
- Understand the inter-dependence of all stakeholders in managing and delivering healthcare services
- Identify ways of enhancing health service user involvement and inter-disciplinary collaboration in your own area of professional practice to enhance collaborative working potential.

Introduction

Since its creation in 1948, the UK National Health Service (NHS) has become increasingly complex and diverse in its provision of health and social care services. Yet despite many innovations, the NHS has failed to keep pace with the changes in society because its systems are too rigid, linear and un-businesslike, resulting in inefficiencies through duplication of services as well as inequalities of service provision (DH 2000a; 2000b; 2005; 2008a).

These inefficiencies are not unique to the UK; health systems around the world may become unsustainable if unchanged over the next 15 years, creating massive financial burdens, as well as health problems, for current and future generations (Pricewaterhouse Coopers 2005). Globally, healthcare is threatened by a confluence of powerful trends – increasing demand, rising costs, fragmented services, disjointed care, poor quality, and misaligned incentives (Kodner 2006).

The UK Government expects care organizations to operate as 'Whole Systems' (DH 2000b, 2005) and become more flexible and businesslike delivering efficient care of a consistently high quality. Whole systems working requires that practitioners within health and social care learn to integrate interprofessional working and user consultation into their daily practice. As such, this chapter will introduce the concept of whole systems working as a model for developing critical and creative practice within health and social care and will discuss its strengths and limitations.

Characteristics of a whole system approach

Hudson et al. (2003: 233) argue that the classic fragmented approach to care, where individual professionals only work within the bounds of their own professional team, is inadequate to deal with the increased 'task scope' facing the modern professional. Whole systems working is a radical way of thinking about change in complex situations and provides a combination of theoretical and practical methods of working across boundaries (Pratt et al. 1999). A 'whole system' is defined as a mix of individuals, professions, services and sites of provision who are collectively concerned with delivering care by working together in a coordinated manner (Hudson 2006). Whole systems working helps people make organizational connections (with people and ideas) that enable them to find sustainable long-term solutions to local concerns (Pratt et al. 1999). This coordinated approach involves integration, and cooperation, in the planning, delivery and evaluation of care. The whole systems approach is therefore concerned with the 'big picture' within complex environments.

It involves:

- Identifying the various components of the whole system – typically the individual, organizations and their functions – and then systematically assessing the nature of the links and relationships between each of these.
- Recognizing the benefits of whole systems working – for example, opportunities to share the costs of investments.
- Understanding the specific risks which arise in adopting a whole systems approach (Lebcir 2006; Pratt et al. 2005).

Integrated care and whole systems working

The whole systems approach emphasizes the importance of person-centred holistic and integrated care planning, with the service user at the core of their care (Kharicha et al. 2004). The needs of the patient are central to the care process and should be in tune with the individual's personal values (Ford and McCormack 2000). It emphasizes the importance of understanding the whole person: personal and developmental issues (for example, feeling emotionally understood) and the context (the family and how life has been affected) (Little et al. 2001). This vision requires health professionals to engage with stakeholders, 'listening to and co-researching with, rather than telling and instructing' (Chapman 2002: 22). It requires an integrated partnership approach to working across health and social care teams and traditional boundaries. A central tenet requires that relationships between all people in the care environment are nurtured (Brooker 2004). A whole systems approach focuses on the positive and strengths of the system and not the negatives and weaknesses (SHARP at: http://www.careplans.co.uk/pcc-key.htm).

Long-term conditions clearly represent a pressing challenge for the NHS, but the problem is growing due to increasing obesity, sedentary lifestyles, and an ageing population. An example of the application of whole systems working was identified in the White Paper *Our Health, Our Care, Our Say: A New Direction for Community Services* (DH 2006a).

There is, then, an expressed understanding on the part of the Department of Health (2006a) that the delivery of care to meet increasingly complex needs should be joined up and that social and healthcare professionals, as well as carers and voluntary services, are important in achieving this. The aim is to improve health outcomes for people with long-term conditions by offering a personalized care plan for vulnerable people; and to reduce emergency bed day usage by 5 per cent by 2008 through improved care delivery in primary care and community settings (DH 2005a). To this end they propose an increase in joint commissioning, and hence integration, of care between primary care trusts and other local authorities. These aims will be achieved through a new model of care that aims to empower and inform patients, and to create prepared and proactive health and social care teams. The process of change is evident in the increasing availability of decision support tools and clinical information systems (e.g. Summary Assessment of Need Tool, (DH 2008b); Picture Archiving and Communications Systems (NHS 2009 at http://www.connectingforhealth.nhs.uk/newsroom/worldview/protti8)). Case and disease management is central, but supported self-care and the promotion of better public health are also crucial. As such a whole system approach to the delivery of care requires an understanding of what is meant by integrated care as well as the role that the individual practitioners play within this system.

Integrated care pathways (ICPs) provide an excellent example of this whole systems working in action. Middleton et al. (2001) describe ICPs as: 'a multidisciplinary outline of anticipated care, placed in an appropriate time-frame, to help a patient with a specific condition or set of symptoms move progressively through a clinical experience to positive outcomes'. ICPs reduce variation in practice and duplication of effort by providing a single tool for the use of any number of care professionals involved in the management of individuals with specific care needs for example.

Despite such examples, there remains much debate about what exactly integrated care means (Lloyd and Wait 2006). The Care Services Improvement Partnership (2008) state that: 'In its most complete form, integration refers to a single system of needs assessment, service commissioning and/or service provision.' At its least complicated it is loose confederations who engage in ad hoc mutually beneficial partnership working (Hudson 1998, cited in Charlesworth 2003: 145).

A whole systems approach to long-term conditions means:

- Employing an interdisciplinary team approach guided by consensus building and mutual respect
- Creation of a shared vision of healthcare that permits each practitioner and the patient to contribute their particular knowledge and skills
- Integration of services through the continuum of care to ensure that patients are treated at the most appropriate level of care and that their journey through the system is efficient
- Integration of clinical expertise such that all specialties, including primary care, are equal members of a multi-specialty team jointly controlling resources
- Financial integration so that all parties in the system (primary care doctors, consultants, and hospitals) are jointly responsible for ensuring that resources are spent effectively
- Integration of leadership and management to ensure partnership between clinical governance and administration in achieving shared goals
- Integration of culture and vision within a single organizational structure dedicated to providing high quality, cost-effective care (Ham et al. 2003; Boon et al. 2004; Light and Dixon 2004).

The role of the individual practitioner within this whole system is important and later in the chapter critical and creative thinking as strategies for working within organic and non-linear whole systems will be developed. It was the collective failings of individuals working outside of the framework of an integrated whole system that were responsible for notable scandals such as the deaths of Victoria Climbié (Laming 2003) and Baby P (Ofsted 2008). Such failings, and many others besides, establish the importance of whole systems.

Enhancing quality in integrated care

Achieving the best care for service users therefore requires that the providers of care work in joined up ways that take full advantage of the range of skills and knowledge available to them from within their own professions and agencies as well as from working collaboratively with other professionals, agencies and individuals, including recipients of care. Lank (2005) refers to this collaborative advantage as working for the benefit of the organization, those involved in the delivery of care and the end user.

Reflective activity 3.1

- In your area of practice how are service users currently consulted about the quality of the service they receive?
- What measures would improve their opportunity to be more involved in the care planning process?
- What resources would you need in your service to strengthen user involvement in evaluating the quality of the care they receive?

Classically the quality of care has been measured by enumerating the numbers of clients seen, operations undertaken and lives saved – things that can be counted. Since the 1990s service commissioners and providers have come to realize that the quality of care is about more than mere outputs and that the 'outcomes of care', which include the way in which the care is experienced, are important. Pinnock and Dimmock (2003) defined outcomes as a process which functions at the individual, service and strategic level while Campbell et al. (2000) suggest that there are two principal dimensions of quality of care: access to, and effectiveness of, both clinical and inter-personal care. Such best value outcomes, Evans (2003: 111) argues, are best achieved within the operation of partnership working, collaboration, a culture of 'appropriate enquiry' and within a learning environment.

Thus quality integrated care has the patient at its heart. This reflects the Department of Health user consultation, involvement and choice agenda (DH 2006b) and initiatives such as the 'expert patient' (DH 2001) and 'direct payments' (The Crown 2003). The proliferation of user consultation has been described as a move from patients being seen as consumers of care to one of democratization and even citizenship (Beresford and Croft 2003).

There are no hard and fast solutions to solving the problems facing health and social care provision in the UK. Most research to date only addresses small elements of care provision, with little hard evidence about how to develop systems which are innovative, flexible and creative enough to meet the challenges of modern healthcare delivery. Whole systems provide a safe environment in which practitioners can develop novel and innovative practice because they have a non-blame culture but instead learn and develop from their collective mistakes. Such systems are open and honest, and practice within them is characterized by the ability to perform not only by examining and applying fact, but also by creating and working with possibilities. Whole systems are responsive to the needs of the individual and because there is agreement between all stakeholders as to the division of roles and responsibilities there are fewer gaps in care provision and the duplication of effort is minimized (DH 2007).

Challenges of implementing a whole systems approach

There are a number of challenges which deflect from the creation and success of whole systems approaches to the delivery of care. Such challenges include:

- Divergent professional identities
- Increasing consumer expectation
- Proliferation in information technologies and communication between health and social care organizations (Chapman 2002)
- Complex health and social care needs of an ageing population
- Current workloads
- Complex and fragmented health and social care organizations which concentrate on getting the job done, rather than on getting the job done well
- Fast changing and unstable environment of care.

Long-established professional identities, roles and ways of working mean that it is hard to see one's own place within a bigger picture, such as whole systems, since classic professional identity plays down doubt, emotions and humility, and tackles head on the challenges that practice presents (Davies 2003).

Moving to whole systems working will doubtless dilute some of the classic power of the professions who increasingly have to work together, engage with new more integrated frameworks of care (e.g. National Service Frameworks) and have to submit themselves to more scrutiny (e.g. Healthcare Commission inspections). This move towards a more integrated, patient-centred process of working requires a change in the mind-set of the professional. Inevitably people resist and fear change (Hopson and Adams 1976) and seek to defend the territory that they regard as being their own (Scottish Centre for Telehealth 2007). Increases in communication technologies and the resultant growth in interactions between organizations and agencies increase the complexity of the working environment (Chapman 2002) and busy practitioners reluctant to engage in time-consuming interactions delay decision-making resulting in a focus on the short-term solutions producing immediate benefits (Senge 1990). See Table 3.1.

Addressing the challenges of implementing a whole systems approach

Overcoming these challenges to developing whole systems approaches to the delivery of health and social care therefore requires that the AP engages with the benefits that new technology can provide (e.g. using the internet to find new sources of knowledge). They need to create networks with

Table 3.1 Characteristics of a whole system compared to a conventional healthcare system

Whole system	Conventional system
Focuses on the client/patient/service user at the centre of the system	Focuses on processes within the organization
Demonstrates evidence of integrated interprofessional working	Evidence of disjointed working often in uniprofessional or multiprofessional ways
Organization is open to continuous learning, adapting and evolving its practices	Driven by policy reform and policy guidance
Demonstrates evidence of creative practice	Demonstrates evidence of resistance to change and is often defensive of current practice
Holistic: considers all aspects of the system as an integrated whole working together	Task orientated: considers the task to be achieved and does not see the whole picture

like-minded individuals to explore new ways of working both from within their own profession and organization and from outside. They should engage with lifelong learning and use supervision, appraisals and personal development planning to enhance their own development and identify and develop their role within the whole system.

The AP working within a whole system needs, therefore to be:

- connected with self and others
- reflective, reflexive and empathetic
- a team player
- cognizant of, and able to call on, the expertise and experience of others (Davies 2003).

In summary then, the central tenet of a whole systems approach requires health professionals to be comfortable with not knowing exactly what the future of health and social care delivery will look like. We need to therefore develop the knowledge and skills to adapt our ways of thinking and working to face the challenges ahead. There is no quick solution or quick fix, no right way of doing things' so what is the answer? On a global scale the answer lies in partnership working, new ways of thinking and problem solving with the patient and local community at the centre. We need to be comfortable with not knowing the answer but having a range of strategies that encourage us to look at the whole picture, think laterally and creatively about how to address the challenges rather than only looking for quick fixes to immediate problems.

Given the complex and adaptive nature of the health and social care environment it is necessary to understand how a complex organization operates. The next section will therefore help to demystify the notion of complexity theory and the health and social care organization as a complex adaptive system (CAS). It will begin to explore the place of the advanced nurse practitioner in a CAS.

Applying complexity theory to whole systems working

While there are many types of 'systems' that exist, it is most common for people to invoke the 'machine' metaphor when thinking about health and social care organizational systems (Morgan 1997).

> The machine metaphor leads to belief on how the 'system' can be improved: If the system is not working as planned, then identify the broken part and replace it. If the system is too costly, then work towards economies of scale. If the system is not working in a coordinated fashion, then tighten the interconnections between parts of the system (Begun et al. 2003: 253).

This mechanistic view of healthcare systems is based on scientific ideas that have increased our understanding of the world by analysing wholes into their component parts. The complexity of organizational life is broken down into a series of manageable problems and tackled separately (Pratt et al. 1999). In a mechanical system, behaviour is sequential with analysis, planning, action and review occurring after one another, feeding into further cycles. Policy and strategy are separated from implementation and the parts of the system can be separated, standardized, optimized and reassembled to improve the efficiency of the whole. As we saw earlier, globally this linear mechanistic approach has hindered rather than helped progress the ability of health and social care organizations to shape and respond to changing societal needs. It is important to understand therefore how we can change this view of how an organization works to develop contemporary understandings of organizational behaviour.

Complex adaptive systems

One such way of understanding organizations is if we think of them as complex living and interconnected adaptive systems (Pratt et al. 1999). Complexity science is concerned with explaining how 'living' systems work (e.g. stock markets, human bodies, organs and cells, trees and hospitals).

In defining a complex adaptive system (CAS), 'complex' implies diversity (Begun et al. 2003). 'Adaptive' suggests the capacity to alter, change and learn from experience (Begun et al. 2003). A 'system' is a set of connected or interdependent things (Senge 1990). In a CAS, the 'things' are independent agents. An agent may be a person, a molecule, a species or an organization, among many others. These agents act based on local knowledge and conditions.

Table 3.2 Core characteristics of complex adaptive systems

- They are nonlinear and dynamic and do not inherently reach fixed-equilibrium points. As a result, system behaviours may appear to be random or chaotic.
- They are composed of independent agents whose behaviours are based on physical, psychological, or social rules rather than the demands of system dynamics.
- Because agents' needs or desires are reflected in their rules, they are not homogeneous, their goals and behaviours are likely to conflict. In response to these conflicts or competitions, agents tend to adapt to each other's behaviours.
- Agents are intelligent. As they experiment and gain experience, agents learn and change their behaviours accordingly. Thus overall system behaviour inherently changes over time.
- Adaptation and learning tend to result in self-organization. Behaviour patterns emerge rather than being designed into the system. The nature of emergent behaviours may range from valuable innovations to unfortunate accidents.
- There is no single point(s) of control. System behaviours are often unpredictable and uncontrollable, and no one is 'in charge.' Consequently, the behaviours of complex adaptive systems can usually be more easily influenced than controlled.

(Rouse 2000)

A central body, master neuron, or hospital chief executive officer, does not control the agent's individual moves. See Table 3.2.

A CAS has a densely connected web of interacting agents, each operating from its own schema, or local knowledge. CASs are dynamic and massively entangled (Kontopolous 1993), emergent, and robust (Eoyang and Berkas 1999; Marion and Bacon 2000). The concern is with the predictability of their behaviour. Some systems, despite constantly changing, do so in a completely regular manner e.g. a clock pendulum. Other systems are more unstable and move further and further away from their starting conditions until/unless stopped. In addition to being numerous and interdependent, parts and variables, and their relationships, can be nonlinear and discontinuous. Small changes in variables can have small impacts at some times, and large impacts under other conditions. Stable and unstable behaviour, as concepts, are part of the traditional repertoire of physical science. What is novel in a CAS is the concept of something in between – chaotic behaviour. Chaos refers to systems which display behaviour which, though it has certain regularities, defies prediction (Gleick 1987).

Systems behaviour, then, may be divided into two zones, plus the boundary between them; the stable zone, where if disturbed, the system returns to its initial state; and the zone of instability, where a small disturbance leads to movement away from the starting point – generating further divergence. Which type of behaviour is exhibited depends on the local conditions: the laws governing behaviour and the relative strengths of positive and negative feedback mechanisms. Under appropriate conditions, systems may operate at the boundary between these zones – a phase transition or the 'edge of chaos'. It is here that they exhibit the sort of instability which this section has been describing – unpredictability of specific behaviour within a predictable general structure of behaviour (Begun et al. 2003).

Applying complexity theory to health and social care organizations

There is no doubt that care delivery organizations are complex, the typical hospital, for example, has staff from dozens of different professionals and non-professional disciplines, support staff, staff visiting from other organizations to do short-term or one-off jobs and voluntary workers. While the end goal of all of the people working within the hospital environment is the care of the patient, the ways in which they contribute to this are often divergent and lack coordination despite the existence of robust and linear systems of control. Health and social care organizations are also subject to constant change and evolution as a result of changes within society, health and social care research and political agendas.

If whole systems, such as health and social care organizations, are to achieve sustainable development they need to adopt some of the possibilities that an understanding of complex adaptive systems offers – that is to say that whole systems must adopt strategies for change and improvement which recognize that the agents within the system are intelligent and that their practice is constantly evolving as a result of education and experience. If the AP is to function as an agent within these emergent systems, they too need to understand their roles within the system and how what they do impacts on other areas of the system.

Despite the complexity and unpredictable nature of change within the CAS, the patient's wishes and needs remain the major influence on how their individual care is delivered. If the whole systems approach to care is in use and as CASs are more amenable to influence than control, interprofessional and inter-agency cooperation are an absolute necessity.

Reflective activity 3.2

Take time out now to list at least six things that would improve interprofessional working in your area of work.

Take time to discuss with colleagues from different disciplines what they value about the job that they do and how they see it contributing to patient care. Ask them what they value about the role that you play in the team and how this helps them achieve their goals.

This need for cooperation leads the argument back to where we started with whole systems approaches to care, that the care has to be integrated, that the delivery of care has to be via interprofessional and interagency working. This collaborative working calls for the agents within the system to recognize that they share some common values and a shared purpose (Hudson et al. 2003).

The traditional barriers of differing professional identities and languages of care remain a real threat. The ANP working within the complex and adapting whole system is, however, endowed with the power to influence how care is delivered, by negotiating shared outcomes of care and showing, by example, that given the adoption of shared goals, there is a real interdependency between professionals. Recognition of this interdependency, and the need for sustainable development mean that practitioners will come to recognize that time spent communicating with other members of the system is time well spent.

Advanced practitioners and complex adaptive systems

The place of the modern health and social care practitioner within the CAS may prove confusing. The central tenet of care delivery is no longer the skills that the individual has to apply to the service user, but the skills they bring to the system in providing care that is negotiated and acted upon with, and not applied to, the service user alongside the core skills of other members of the CAS.

The system within which the advanced practitioner now works is more complex and it may prove difficult for them to recognize the importance of their contribution within this system. As with the more conventional General Systems Theory, however, each individual within a system contributes towards making the system what it is (von Bertalanffy 1971).

Reflective activity 3.3

- What 'systems' do you belong to?
- How do you think they interact and affect each other?
- Can your behaviour in one system be explained by the impact on you of another system?
- Can you control the behaviour in one system and change the behaviour of another?

The importance of creative thinking in whole systems working

Perhaps most importantly in today's information age, thinking skills are viewed as crucial for educated persons to cope with a rapidly changing world. Many believe that specific knowledge will not be as important to tomorrow's workers and citizens as the ability to learn and make sense of new information.

(Gough 1991, cited in Edgar et al. 2008)

In order to deal effectively with complex change, Simpson and Courtenay (2002) suggest that APs must become skilled in higher level critical thinking, problem solving and creative thinking abilities. These skills enable APs to extend their knowledge and understanding while challenging their own assumptions, values and beliefs and how these interface with the cultural norms of their clinical practice. This section will discuss the concept of creative thinking and explore strategies that can help the AP to develop creative thinking skills. The relationship between critical and creative thinking will first be explored.

Understanding the relationship between critical and creative thinking

Critical and creative thinking are complementary skills which co-occur to varying degrees in a wide range of thinking tasks. Both types of thinking are essential to effective whole systems working in order to become more efficient at appraising the evidence we use to make judgements about quality, be comfortable with changing political and organizational landscapes, and innovate in health and social care delivery. In an activity like problem solving both critical and creative thinking are important. First, we must analyse the problem; then we must generate possible solutions; next we must choose and implement the best solution; and finally, we must evaluate the effectiveness of the solution.

The most commonly cited consensus definition of critical thinking acknowledges that it is 'a purposeful, self-regulatory judgement' (APA 1990) as described in Chapter 1. L'Eplattenier (2001) found most definitions of critical thinking describe it as two-dimensional. The cognitive dimension consists of reflective, reasoned thinking and the affective dimension consists of an inquisitive spirit and open-mindedness to divergent perspectives (L'Eplattenier 2001). Critical thinking is logical and convergent, narrowing down to unique answers or a small number of ideas which can be further analysed and implemented. (Marzano et al. 1987, cited by Vardi 1999; Nickerson 1987; Scriven and Paul 1996).

Creative thinking, on the other hand, is the ability to think about something in novel or unusual ways, or to process already known information to come up with unique insights or solutions to problems that are original, imaginative and uncommon (de Bono 1978; Ruggiero 1988). Creative thinking has been categorized as something we are born with but the literature acknowledges that it can be developed through activities and teaching strategies. Creative thinking starts from the description of the problem, and diverges to give many ideas, or possible answers, for solving it, (Santrock 2004). In effect, critical thinking produces solutions, and creative thinking produces ideas – large numbers of them – from which the solution can be selected.

Van Hook and Tegano (2002: 1) define creativity as 'an interpersonal and intrapersonal process by means of which original high quality and genuinely significant products are developed'. The act of creativity can be performed by an individual, a group, or an organization – or all of these working together – to produce a creative outcome, to achieve innovation, profits, quality, knowledge, or some other desired result. Edwards (2001: 222) adds that creativity 'involves the openness to ideas and the willingness to encourage the exploration of the unknown even if not easily manageable'. Creativity also includes a wide range of interpretations and beliefs based on an individual's personal style and experiences (Edgar et al. 2008). In health and social care the three core components of creativity are expertise, motivation and creative thinking skills.

Expertise involves intellectual, technical and procedural knowledge (Benner 1984). The internal motivation and passion to solve the problem at hand can lead to solutions which are far more creative than external rewards which may be financial (Jones-Devitt and Smith 2007). In turn, creative thinking skills determine how flexibly and imaginatively people approach problems (de Bono 2007).

One cornerstone of advanced practice is to find the connections between critical and creative thinking so that thinking becomes holistic (Ruggiero 1988). In this way both the production and evaluation of ideas can be developed. Within such an holistic framework, a connection can be made between thinking abilities or dispositions, attitudes and values, skills and processes. According to Ruggiero (1988) and Oxman-Michelli (1992, cited in Vardi 1999), certain dispositions, also referred to as a 'critical spirit', facilitate and make the thinking process effective. Table 3.3 provides examples of different types of dispositions considered essential to effective thinking. Critical thinking and

Table 3.3 Examples of dispositions considered necessary for critical and creative thinking

Critical thinking	Creative thinking
Interest in sources of attitudes, beliefs and values	Reject standardized formats for problem solving
Eagerness to develop mental processes	Have an interest in a wide range of related and divergent fields
Willingness to make mistakes	Self-confidence and intellectual autonomy
Positive attitude toward novelty	
Interest in widening experience	Curiosity and attentiveness
Passion for truth	Enthusiasm and perseverance
Ruggiero (1988: 28)	Objectivity, integrity and humility
	Fairmindedness, readiness to listen and consider others' points of view
	Use trial-and-error methods in their experimentation
	Are future orientated
	Oxman-Michelli (1992, cited in Vardi 1999)

creativity lead to critical practice. That is the delivery of care that is based on a system of thought that engages evidence from many sources including research, personal and shared experience, interprofessional experience, the user's view point, ethics, policy and reality. Brechin (2000) states that the critical practitioner utilizes 'analysis, action and reflexivity', they 'respect others as equals' 'adopt an open and "not knowing" [enquiring] approach to practice' and take time to understand themselves and others while forging useful working relationships.

Reflective activity 3.4   Exploring your professional values

Take time now to reflect on the values that underpin your professional practice to understand how that influences the way in which you approach and solve problems.

- What brought you into, and keeps you in, your specialist field of practice?
- Who and what has influenced your career choices and practice? How?
- What are the sources of satisfaction and dissatisfaction in practice?
- What has influenced your understanding of 'illness' and what are the underlying assumptions in this understanding?
- What skills, knowledge and characteristics define your practice?
- How has your view of practice and your role developed over the course of your career and why?
- How might users of your service view your specialist field of practice?

A wide range of skills in both critical, and creative, thinking are identified in the literature (see Table 3.4). Examination of these skills shows the difficulties that can arise when attempting to separate these two 'types' of thinking. Under the headings of both 'critical' and 'creative' thinking are listed similar skills. For instance 'restructuring' appears similar in nature to 'finding relevant connections and combining information'. At other times, the two skill lists highlight differences as to when to apply seemingly contradictory skills such as 'judging' on the one hand, and 'deferring judgement' on the other.

Reflective activity 3.5   Analysis of a practice issue

Take time here to reflect on a problem or issue that you have faced recently in your practice by completing the following activity.

- Choose a practice problem or issue
- How is the problem constructed in the practice setting?
- What is the history of this construction and the social and cultural values that support this construction?
- What are the healthcare practices in response to the problem?
- What knowledge underpins these practices and whose interests do they serve?

- What structures are maintaining the current situation?
- What needs to be done to improve the service/practice?
- Who are the key players that need to be involved in finding a solution to the problem?

Table 3.4 Examples of skills used in critical and creative thinking

Critical thinking	Creative thinking
From Ennis (1987, cited in Vardi 1999: 457)	From Lubart (1994, cited in Vardi 1999: 459)
Focussing on a question	Problem finding
Analysing arguments	Problem definition
Judging the credibility of a source	Problem representation
Observing and judging observation reports	Strategy selection
Deducing and judging deductions	Noticing relevant new information
Inducing and judging inductions	Comparing disparate information
Making value judgements	Finding relevant connections and
Defining and judging definitions	combining information
Identifying assumptions	Generating multiple ideas
From Marzano et al. (1988, cited in Vardi 1999: 458)	From Ruggiero (1988: 28)
Comparing	Deferring judgement
Classifying	Shifting perspective
Ordering	Generating imaginative ideas
Representing	
Summarizing	From De Bono (1978: 50)
Restructuring	Generating new ideas
Predicting	Challenging assumptions
Elaborating	Generating alternatives
Identifying attributes, relationships, main ideas, errors	

Models of creative thinking

While some models make it appear that creativity is a somewhat magical process, the predominant models lean more toward the theory that novel ideas emerge from the conscious effort to balance analysis and imagination. The creative process was outlined by Graham Wallas in *The Art of Thought* (1926). He believed that the creative process consisted of five stages which are widely cited in contemporary literature:

1. **Orientation.** As a first step, the problem must be defined and important dimensions identified.

2. **Preparation.** In the second stage, creative thinkers saturate themselves with as much information pertaining to the problem as possible.
3. **Incubation.** Most major problems produce a period during which all attempted solutions will have proved futile. At this point, problem solving may proceed on a subconscious level. While the problem seems to have been set aside, it is still 'cooking' in the background.
4. **Illumination.** The stage of incubation is often ended by a rapid insight or series of insights. These produce the 'Aha!' experience, often depicted in cartoons as a light bulb appearing over the thinker's head.
5. **Verification.** The final step is to test and critically evaluate the solution obtained during the stage of illumination. If the solution proves faulty, the thinker reverts to the stage of incubation, inquiry, observation, expression.

Rossman (1931, cited in Plsek 1996) examined the creative process via questionnaires completed by 710 inventors and expanded Wallas' original five steps to seven (see Table 3.5).

Table 3.5 Adapted from: Rossman's Creativity Model (1931 cited in Plsek 1996).

1. Observe problem
2. Analyse the problem
3. Identify all available information
4. Devise objective solutions
5. Critically analyse solutions for pros and cons
6. Invent new idea
7. Refine final solution

While Rossman still shrouds the 'birth of the new idea' in mystery, his steps leading up to and following this moment of illumination are clearly analytical.

Alex Osborn (1953, cited in Plsek 1996, see Table 3.6), the developer of brainstorming, embraced a similar theory of balance between analysis and imagination in his seven-step model for creative thinking.

Table 3.6 Osborn's Seven-Step Model for Creative Thinking (cited in Plsek 1996)

1. **Orientation:** identify and pick out the salient points of the problem
2. **Preparation:** gather and analyse relevant information
3. **Analysis:** break down the information into relevant pieces
4. **Ideation:** create alternative solutions
5. **Incubation:** allow ideas to ferment
6. **Synthesis:** put the ideas back together
7. **Evaluation:** judge the ideas that emerge.

Common themes behind the models of the creative process

While there are many models for the process of creative thinking, it is not difficult to see the consistent themes that span them all.

The creative process involves purposeful analysis, imaginative idea generation, and critical evaluation – the total creative process is a balance of imagination and analysis.

Older models tend to imply that creative ideas result from subconscious processes, largely outside the control of the thinker. Modern models tend to imply purposeful generation of new ideas, under the direct control of the thinker.

The total creative process requires a drive to action and the implementation of ideas. We must do more than simply imagine new things; we must work to make them concrete realities (Plsek 1996).

Plsek's (1997) model entitled the Directed Creativity Cycle (Figure 3.1) is a synthesis model of creative thinking that combines the concepts behind the various models proposed over the last 80 years.

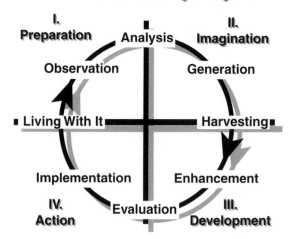

Figure 3.1 Plsek's (1997) Directed Creativity Cycle. © 1997 Paul E Plsek: reproduced with kind permission.

He argues that creative thinking begins with careful observation of the world coupled with thoughtful analysis of how things work and fail. These mental processes create a store of concepts in our memories which we can use to generate novel ideas to meet specific needs by actively searching for associations among concepts. There are many specific techniques that we can use to make these associations; for example, analogies, branching out from a given concept, using a random word, classic brainstorming, and so on. It is not the choice of technique that is important; making the effort to actively search for associations is. The aim is to harvest and further enhance our ideas before we subject them to a final, practical evaluation. But, it is not enough just to have creative thoughts; ideas have no value until we put in the work to implement them. Every new idea that is put into practice changes the world we live in, which re-starts the cycle of observation and analysis. Directed creativity simply means that we make purposeful mental movements to avoid the pitfalls associated with our cognitive mechanisms at each step of this process of searching for novel and useful ideas (Plsek 1996).

Using creative thinking methods to help with problem solving at work

One of the biggest challenges in developing creative thinking is how to free our minds of the built-up patterns we use to enable us to simplify and cope with a complex world. These patterns are based on our past successful experiences in life, education and work. We look at 5x5 and automatically come up with the answer of 25 in our heads. These thinking patterns help us to perform routine tasks rapidly and accurately (e.g. driving). They do, however, make it difficult for us to come up with new ideas and creative solutions to problems, especially when presented with unusual data. So how can we develop our creative thinking skills and abilities?

There are a range of tools and methods that can be used to promote creative thinking and a small selection are presented here.

Tools for defining problems

Rudyard Kipling used a series of questions to help trigger ideas and solve problems. They work because they are short and direct and the 'what' can be applied to many different situations making them a flexible resource. One approach to this is to use the questions in a particular order to guide you through a sequence of thought towards a complete answer:

- What is the problem?
- Where is it happening?
- Why is it happening?
- When is it happening?
- How can you overcome this problem?
- Who do you need to get involved?
- When will you know you have solved the problem?

The first step in solving a creative problem is to define the problem; this may seem obvious yet many creative efforts fail because the problem is unclear or focused in the wrong area. The way in which the problem is stated is half the problem and half the solution. Once you have identified a good problem statement, sometimes the solution is so obvious that, you need little, if any, creative thought afterwards.

Finally the Challenge Method can be used to force oneself, or other people, out of a thinking rut. It can be used to test out ideas for validity and to challenge the problem or situation you are considering when initially defining the problem. One way in which we deal with the complexity of the world is to make assumptions about many things. This pattern-matching ability is a great help in allowing us to take short cuts but limits our capacity to notice things. Thus if we do not take deliberate and conscious action, many things will go by unnoticed.

Reflective activity 3.6

Select all or part of a problem domain you are going to challenge. It may be something that you are finding particularly hard to be creative around.

Find something to challenge and question it deeply. Look at the following in particular:

- Concepts – and broad ideas
- Assumptions – and beliefs that are not questioned
- Boundaries – which you do not yet cross
- Impossibilities – things that it is assumed cannot happen or cannot be done
- 'Essentials' – things you assume cannot be disposed of
- 'Sacred Cows' – things that cannot be challenged.

A useful tool to assist with individual and team decision-making designed by de Bono (1986) is the 'Six Thinking Hats'. This strategy is creative, non-adversarial and cooperative. It forces the individual, or the team to look at a situation from more than one side. Each hat has a colour which represents a perspective that what de Bono called the 'players' can take. The advanced practitioner can use these to aid them in creative and critical thinking which they can use to problem solve and innovate. See Table 3.7.

Challenges associated with developing creative thinking in whole systems work

As we have seen, many of the local and global challenges facing health and social care today are embedded in interconnected systems. Addressing these challenges means moving beyond the limitations of the perspectives, methods and tools of traditional reductionist science and linear management systems. Whole systems thinking (WST) involves looking at systems holistically in order to solve problems. When entire systems are examined, and changes implemented and evaluated, the overall effectiveness of the process,

Table 3.7 de Bono's (1986) Six Thinking Hats

Hat colour	Explanation	Characteristic statements
White	White is neutral – ignore arguments and proposals. Examine only the facts, figures and information. Identify what information is needed and how to get it.	What information do we have? What information is missing? What information do we need? How are we going to get it?
Red	Red is for feelings, hunches and intuition. It allows people to put forward feelings without needing to apologize or justify. Intuition may arise out of experience, and can be valuable, even if not explained.	I feel that it won't work. I don't like how this is being done. My intuition tells me this process isn't sustainable.
Black	Black is negative logical, cautious and critical. It is the most used hat, and arguably the most valuable. It is easy to overuse and stifle creative ideas.	Policy will prevent us from doing that. We don't have the resources. The team doesn't have the needed experience.
Yellow	Yellow is for the optimistic and positive logical view. It looks for how something can be done. It looks for logical benefits.	That might work if we rework the timings. The team could take this further in a second project. We have the resources.
Green	Green is for creativity. New ideas and alternatives. Lateral thinking and other creative techniques are engaged.	We need new ideas. What are the alternatives? Can we do this another way? Is there another explanation?
Blue	Blue is the thinking overview, or process control hat. It is used by the chairperson of the meeting, sets the agenda for thinking, suggests the next step, and asks for summaries, conclusions and decisions.	We have spent far too much time looking for someone to blame. Could we have a summary of your views? I think we should take a look at the priorities.

business, or organization improves dramatically. One small change often solves multiple problems and increases efficiency and performance.

Korten (1995: 11) suggests that whole systems thinking calls for:

a scepticism of simplistic solutions, a willingness to seek out connections between problems and events that conventional discourse ignores, and the courage to delve into subject matter that may lie outside our direct experience and expertise.

The challenge with adopting a whole systems approach to thinking which incorporates critical and creative thinking skills is that little is currently known about how 'best' to reorganize care services and the evidence that we have does not provide a holistic picture of the most effective way to plan and move forwards with certainty. The normal behavioural stance for us, as health professionals, is that prior to taking action we like to feel that we know the truth. However, this cannot always be the case; therefore, our actions are often based on minimizing risk.

Dealing with uncertainty requires special management skills. While it is always commendable to seek the truth, we also need to be able to act on half-truths and uncertainties. De Bono argues (2007) that some people are excellent at managing in situations when things are going very well. There are also people who succeed in managing when things are going badly. Not many people can manage successfully in times of great uncertainty. It is difficult to make plans and decisions when the present is uncertain, it requires a high level of management skill. What is clear, however, is that we cannot rely on traditional reductionist ways of thinking to help guide our plans to reorganize health services. We therefore need to be aware of how uncertainty influences the ways in which we behave and limits our ability to embrace change and think laterally about the bigger picture. Being aware of how our current behaviours limit our actions and tendencies to fall back on traditional safeguards enables us to think more positively about the future. We therefore need to think about the future as a range of 'possibilities'. As de Bono (2007) asserts, 'Possible' might describe something that is low in probability. However, 'possibility' enlarges your perception (and choices); probability narrows them (de Bono 2007).

The challenge for health and social care organizations is to adopt organizational cultures that:

- support creativity and innovation;
- see risk taking as acceptable;
- provide employees with access to sources of knowledge;
- encourage new ideas and ways of doing things;
- allow a free flow of information;
- reward innovation; and
- support good ideas.

Developing critical and creative thinking skills enables the developing AP to examine their management and leadership skills to look at all possibilities when considering explanations that will enable service redesign, effective change management and ultimately the delivery of a high quality care.

Summary

This chapter has established that we work in uncertain times. The political and social climate in which health and social care is practised is one of shifting sands which makes it difficult for the advanced practitioner to understand where they fit into the bigger picture. The argument for a whole systems approach to the delivery of care has been advanced as one potential solution to the development of high quality, responsive and inclusive health and social care. The achievement of high quality outcomes for health and social care require that the practitioner works interprofessionally, focuses on the service user, and engages in creative and critical thinking. Such a move requires that the practitioner questions and is sure about their own value base, that they take time to reflect on the care that they give, that they think creatively and critically and that they are open to change.

Critical and creative thinking has been advanced as a potential solution to overcoming the praxis that exists in the practice setting where the practitioner faces the challenge of delivering fact-based care, but finds that what is already known does not always fit the situation, or that there are uncertainties, ambiguities or as yet unknown factors at play. A range of strategies have been presented to help the AP to develop their creative and critical thinking skills. APs require the ability to check assumptions, challenge the rules that bind them to acting only on certainties, engage their imagination and intuition, take risks, understand how their values, beliefs, education and experience can constrain their thinking and their ability to solve problems in creative ways in order to free their minds to embrace their full creative potential.

Key points

- Modern health and social care delivery is increasingly complex.
- Standard linear models of managing care delivery are failing to keep pace with the modernization agenda.
- The whole systems (non-linear) approach to care delivery is one potential route to achieving modern health and social care delivery.
- Whole systems require that practitioners are creative and critical in their thinking.
- Whole systems value the client's viewpoint and the contribution of all members of the organization.
- Creative and critical thinkers working within whole systems are capable of delivering high quality outcomes for and with their clients.

References

American Philosophical Association (1990) *Critical Thinking: A Statement of Expert Consensus*. The Delphi Report. Committee on Pre-College Philosophy. ERIC No. ED315–423. Millbrae: APA.

Begun, J.W., Zimmerman, B. and Dooley, K. (2003) Healthcare organisations as complex adaptive systems, in S.M. Mick and M. Wyttenbach (eds) *Advances in Health Care Organization Theory*. San Francisco: Jossey-Bass.

Benner, P. (1984). *From Novice to Expert: Excellence and power in clinical nursing practice.* Menlo Park: Addison-Wesley.

Beresford, P. and Croft, S. (2003) Involving service users in management: citizenship, access and rapport, in J. Reynolds, J. Henderson, J. Seden, J. Charlesworth and A. Bullman (eds) *The Managing Care Reader: A reader.* London: Routledge.

Boon, H., Verhoef, M., O'Hara, D. and Findlay, B. (2004) From parallel practice to integrative health care: a conceptual framework. *BMC Health Services Research*, 4: 15. www.biomedcentral.com/1472–6963/4/15 (accessed 21 January 2009).

Brechin, A. (2000) Introducing critical practice, in A. Brechin, H. Brown and M. Eby (eds) *Critical Practice in Health and Social Care.* London: Sage.

Brooker, D. (2004) What is person-centred care in dementia? *Reviews in Clinical Gerontology*, 13: 215–22.

Campbell, S.M., Roland, M.O. and Buetow, S.A. (2000) Defining quality of care. *Social Science and Medicine* 51(11): 1611–25.

Care Services Improvement Partnership (2008) *Bringing the NHS and Local Government Together: A practical guide to integrated working.* www.icn.csip.org.uk/practicalguidetointegratedworking (accessed 16 January 2009).

Chapman, J. (2002) *System Failure: Why governments must learn to think differently.* London: Demos, p. 22.

Charlesworth, J. (2003) Managing across professional and agency boundaries, in J. Seden and J. Reynolds *Managing Care in Context.* London: Routledge.

Davies, C. (2003) Workers, professions and identity, in J. Henderson and D. Atkinson *Managing Care in Context.* London: Routledge.

De Bono, E. (1978) *Teaching Thinking.* Harmondsworth: Penguin, p. 50.

De Bono, E. (1986) *Six Thinking Hats.* New York: Little Brown.

De Bono, E. (2007) *How to Have Creative Ideas.* London: Vermillion.

Department of Health (DH) (2000a) *The NHS Plan: A plan for investment, a plan for reform.* London: DH.

Department of Health (DH) (2000b) *A Quality Strategy for Social Care 2000.* London: DH.

Department of Health (DH) (2001) *The Expert Patient: A new approach to chronic disease management for the 21st century.* London: DH.

Department of Health (DH) (2005) *Creating a Patient-led NHS: Delivering the NHS Improvement Plan.* London: DH.

Department of Health (DH) (2006a) *Our Health, our Care, our Say: A new direction for community services.* London: DH.

Department of Health (DH) (2006b) *Reward and Recognition: The principles and practice of service user payment and reimbursement in health and social care,* 2nd edn. London: DH.

Department of Health (DH) (2008a) *High Quality Care for All: NHS Next Stage Review final report.* London: DH.

Department of Health (DH) (2008b) *Integrated Packages Approach to Care (InPAC) CDST Clinical Decision Support Tool (Adults of Working Age and Older People Mental Health Services) (Version 2).* London: DH.

Edgar, D.W., Faulkner, P., Franklin, E. et al. (2008) *Creative Thinking: opening up a world of thought. Techniques*: 46–49. www.acteonline.org (accessed 16 January 2009).

Edwards, S.M. (2001) The technology paradox: efficiency versus creativity. *Creativity Research Journal*, 13: 221–8.

Ennis, R.H. (1987) A taxonomy of critical thinking dispositions and abilities. Cited by: Vardi, I. (1999) Critical and creative thinking: How can it be fostered and developed at the tertiary level?, in K. Martin, N. Stanley and N. Davison (eds) *Teaching in the Disciplines/Learning in Context*, 457. Proceedings of the 8th Annual Teaching

Learning Forum, The University of Western Australia, February 1999. Perth: UWA. http://lsn.curtin.edu.au/tlf/tlf1999/vardi.html

Eoyang, G.H. and Berkas, T.H. (1999) Evaluating performance in a complex, adaptive system CAS, in M.R. Lissak H.P. and Gunz (eds) *Managing Complexity in Organizations: A View in Many Directions.* Westport, CT: Quorum.

Evans, M. (2003) The quest for quality: reflecting on the modernisation agenda, in J. Reynolds, J. Henderson, J. Seden A. and Bullman (eds) *The Managing Care Reader.* London: Routledge.

Ford, P. and McCormack, B. (2000) Keeping the person in the centre of nursing. *Nursing Standard,* 14(46): 40–4.

Gleick, J. (1987) *Chaos: Making a New Science.* New York: Viking Penguin.

Gough, D. (1991) Thinking about thinking. Alexandria, Virginia. National Association of Elementary School Principals, in D.W. Edgar et al. (2008) *Creative Thinking: Opening Up a World of Thought. Techniques: 46–49.* www.acteonline.org (accessed 21 Jan 2009).

Ham, C., York, N., Sutch, S. and Shaw, R. (2003) Hospital bed utilisation in the NHS, Kaiser Permanente, and the US Medicare programme: analysis of routine data. *British Medical Journal,* 327: 1257–61.

Hopson, B. and Adams, J. (1976) Towards an understanding of transition, in J. Adams, B. Hopson and H. Hayes (eds) *Transition: Understanding and Managing Personal Change.* London: Martin Robertson and Co.

Hudson, B. (2006) Policy change and policy dilemmas: interpreting the community services White Paper in England (2006). *International Journal of Integrated Care,* www.ijic.org: 1568–4156 (accessed 21 January 2009).

Hudson, B., Hardy, B., Henwood, M. and Wistow, G. (2003) In pursuit of inter-agency collaboration in the public sector: what is the contribution of theory and research?, in J. Reynolds, J. Henderson, J. Seden, and A. Bullman (eds) *The Managing Care Reader: A reader.* London: Routledge.

Jones-Devitt, S. and Smith, L. (2007) *Critical Thinking and Social Care.* London: Sage.

Kharicha, K., Levin, E., Iliffe, S. and Davey, B. (2004) Social work, general practice and evidence based policy in the collaborative care of older people: current problems and future possibilities. *Health and Social Care in the Community,* 12: 134–41.

Kodner, D.L. (2006) Whole-system approaches to health and social care partnerships for the frail elderly: an exploration of North American models and lessons. *Health and Social Care in the Community,* 14(5): 384–90.

Kontopolous, K. (1993) *The Logic of Social Structure.* New York: Cambridge University Press.

Korten, D.C. (1995) *When Corporations Rule the World.* London: Earthscan Publications.

Laming, W.H. (2003) *The Victoria Climbié Inquiry: Report of an inquiry.* www.victoria-climbie-inquiry.org.uk/finreport/finreport.htm (accessed 16 January 2009).

Lank, E. (2005) *Collaborative Advantage: How organisations win by working together.* London: Palgrave Macmillan.

Lebcir, R. (2006) *Healthcare Management: The contribution of systems thinking.* https://uhra.herts.ac.uk/dspace/bitstream/2299/683/1/S65.pdf (accessed: 21 January 2009).

L'Éplattenier, N. (2001) Tracing the development of critical thinking in baccalaureate nursing students. *Journal of the New York State Nurses Association,* 32(2): 27–32.

Light, D. and Dixon, M. (2004) Making the NHS more like Kaiser Permanente. *British Medical Journal,* 328: 763–5.

Little, P., Everitt, H., Williamson, I. et al. (2001) Preferences of patients for patient centred approach to consultation in primary care: observational study. *British Medical Journal,* 322: 468–75.

Lloyd, J. and Wait, S. (2006) *Integrated Care: A guide for policy makers*. London: Alliance for Health and the Future.

Marion, R. and Bacon, J. (2000) Organizational extinction and complex systems. *Emergence*, 1(4): 71–96.

Middleton, S., Barnett, J. and Reeves, D. (2001) What is an integrated Care Pathway? http://www.medicine.ox.ac.uk/bandolier/painres/download/whatis/What_is_an_ICP. pdf (accessed 26 September 2009).

Morgan, G. (1997) *Images of Organization* 2nd edn. Thousand Oaks, CA: Sage.

National Health Service (2009) *Connecting for Health*. http://www.connectingforhealth. nhs.uk/newsroom/worldview/protti8 (accessed 9 February 2009).

Nickerson, R.S. (1987) Dimensions of thinking: a critique, in B.F. Jones and L. Idol (eds), *Dimensions of Thinking and Cognitive Instruction*. Hillsdale: Lawrence Erlbaum Associates, Publishers.

Ofsted, Healthcare Commission and HM inspectorate of Constabulary (2008) Joint Area Review: Haringey Children's Services Authority Area. www.ofsted.gov.uk/ oxcare_providers/la_download/(id)/4657/(as)/JAR/jar_2008_309_fr.pdf (accessed 16 January 2009).

Pinnock, M. and Dimmock, B. (2003) Managing for outcomes, in J. Henderson and D. Atkinson *Managing Care in Context*. London: Routledge.

Plsek, P.E. (1996) *Working Paper: Models for the creative process*. www. directedcreativity.com/pages/WPModels.html (accessed 16 January 2009).

Plsek, P.E. (1997) *Creativity, Innovation, and Quality*. Milwaukee, WI: ASQ Quality Press.

Pratt, J., Gordon, P. and Plampling, D. (1999) *Working Whole Systems: Putting theory into practice in organisations*. London: Kings Fund.

Pratt, J., Gordon, P., Plampling, D. and Wheatley, M.J. (2005) *Working Whole Systems: Putting theory into practice in organisations*, 2nd edn. Oxford: Radcliffe Medical Press.

Pricewaterhouse Coopers (2005) *Healthcast 2020: Creating a sustainable future*. London: Pricewaterhouse Coopers LLP. http://pwchealth.com/cgi-local/hregister.cgi? link=reg/hc2020en.pdf 9 (accessed 16 January 2009).

Rouse, W.B. (2000) Managing complexity: disease control as a complex adaptive system. *Information Knowledge Systems Management,* 2(2): 143–65.

Ruggiero, V.R. (1988) *Teaching Thinking across the Curriculum*. New York: Harper and Row Publishers.

Santrock, J.W. (2004) *Educational Psychology* 2nd edn. Upper Saddle River, NJ: Allyn and Bacon.

Scottish Centre for Telehealth (2007) *Delivering Better Outcomes through Better Partnerships: A case of mutual dependency*. Scottish Centre for Telehealth Annual Conference, 21 November 2007. www.sct.scot.nhs.uk/documents/MikeMartin. ppt#1 (accessed 16 January 2009).

Scriven, M. and Paul, R. (1996). *Defining Critical Thinking*. http://www.sonoma.edu/ CThink/University/univclass/Defining.nclk [24 Jan 1999] (accessed 16 January 2009).

Senge, P.M. (1990) *The Fifth Discipline: The art and practice of the learning organization*. London: Random House Business Books.

SHARP at: http://www.careplans.co.uk/pcc-key.htm (accessed 16 January 2009).

Simpson, E. and Courtenay, M. (2002) Critical thinking in nursing education: Literature review. *International Journal of Nursing Practice*, 8: 89–98.

The Crown (2003) The Community Care, Services for Carers and Children's Services (Direct Payments) (England) Regulations 2003. www.opsi.gov.uk/si/si2003/ 20030762.htm (accessed 16 January 2009).

Van Hook, C.W. and Tegano, D.W. (2002) The relationship between creativity and conformity among preschool children, *Journal of Creative Behaviour*, 36: 1–16.

Vardi, I. (1999). Critical and creative thinking: How can it be fostered and developed at the tertiary level?, in K. Martin, N. Stanley and N. Davison (eds) *Teaching in the Disciplines/Learning in Context*, 455–461. Proceedings of the 8th Annual Teaching Learning Forum, The University of Western Australia, February 1999. Perth: UWA. http://lsn.curtin.edu.au/tlf/tlf1999/vardi.html (accessed 16 January 2009).

Von Bertalanffy, L. (1971) *General Systems Theory: Foundations, Development, application*. London: Allen Lane.

Wallas, G. (1926) *The Art of Thought*. New York: Harcourt Brace.

World Health Organization (WHO) (2003) *The World Health Report 2003: Shaping the future*. Geneva: WHO.

4 Lifelong learning in judgement and decision-making

Mooi Standing and Antonio Sama

Overview

This chapter explores the importance and characteristics of lifelong learning in the development of professional identity, expertise and clinical judgement and decision-making skills in health and social care. It discusses different forms of tacit and explicit professional knowledge and skills and methods of acquiring, enhancing and applying them to clinical practice. The important contribution and characteristics of effective informal, work-based learning are discussed together with strategies to make formal, interprofessional university-based continuing professional development programmes participative and relevant in transforming clinical practice. Reflective activities are included to enable readers to relate issues to developing clinical judgement/decision-making skills.

Objectives

- Relate judgement and decision-making to professional identity and expertise
- Understand different forms of tacit/explicit knowledge and methods of lifelong learning
- Describe how mentoring/supervision helps to develop judgement/decision-making skills
- Describe principles of an interprofessional peer learning community to transform practice
- Identify tactics to maximize informal learning opportunities in judgement/decision-making
- Identify tactics to maximize formal learning opportunities in judgement/decision-making

Introduction

The application of whole systems and complexity theory to the organization and delivery of health and social care in the United Kingdom (Chapter 3) highlights the effects of radical changes in social policy with far-reaching implications for professional practice and lifelong learning. For example, reforming healthcare and social services may be associated with addressing perceived threats to the continued viability of the welfare state (Kemshall 2002), as follows:

- **Loss of legitimacy:** Professional authority and expertise are not taken for granted and are challenged more, for example, 'the existing armamentarium of theories and techniques applied by professionals to remove the troubles that beset society has no longer public confidence' (Schön 1983: 11). This is exacerbated by reports of tragedies in which health and social care professionals and organizations are perceived to have failed to deliver appropriate care and/or ensure adequate protection of vulnerable patients or clients (Alaszewski 2001). This has contributed to greater public accountability of health/social care professionals for their actions.
- **Spiralling costs:** Demographic changes, such as an ageing population, contribute to an increasing demand for services coinciding with a declining productive workforce needed to generate wealth to fund health and social care. The effects of the recent global financial crisis exacerbate the problem, and encourage those who can afford it to pay for private healthcare. The capacity of the welfare state to sustain a 'safety net' in meeting public health and social care needs in times of adversity is being questioned by observations that 'risk is replacing need as the core principle of social policy formation and welfare delivery' (Kemshall 2002: 1).
- **Inefficiency:** Public services are perceived as inefficient compared to commercial businesses resulting in a modernization agenda that began in the 1980s by a Conservative government led by Margaret Thatcher and continued by a New Labour government led by Tony Blair. This is associated with introducing a more competitive market culture and reframing patients or clients as consumers of services. This implies they will have more choice and enjoy higher quality, well-coordinated and standardized systems (Mintzberg 1979) of health and social care. However, Purdy (1999: 74) questions whether health is perceived as 'a right of citizenship, guaranteed by the welfare state' or as 'a duty of citizenship' to be socially responsible, adopt a healthy lifestyle to prevent healthcare problems, and alleviate the strain on the welfare state. It is evidently more efficient to prevent disease than deal with its effects but clinical judgement and decision-making are usually associated with secondary care as opposed to primary preventative care. Practitioners are, therefore, obliged to give health promotion advice regarding future self-care.

Health and social care professionals are, therefore, required to continually demonstrate a high level of clinical competence, be accountable for their actions, utilize precious resources efficiently, and promote prevention in a challenging and constantly changing socio-politico-economic context.

As such, it is very important to understand and enhance health/social care professionals' lifelong learning in developing and adapting expertise according to the prevailing demands of social policy, NHS reforms, and public expectations. Initial and continuing professional development is associated with a gradual transition from novice (behaviour assumed to be based on adherence to rules) to expert (behaviour assumed to be based on intuitive understanding) and progress is influenced by the culture of the clinical environment in which experience is gained aided (Schön 1983; Dreyfus and Dreyfus 1986; Boak and Thompson 1998; Jasper 2003). The challenge is how to enhance situated (practice-centred) lifelong learning to develop practitioners' professional identity and clinical judgement and decision-making skills in the ever changing setting of health and social care (Gherardi and Nicolini 2002; Taylor 2006: 1200). It requires an understanding of the nature of professional knowledge and ways of learning, including informal work-based learning and formal university-based continuing professional development programmes.

Encoded, embodied, embrained and embedded knowledge

Lifelong learning in the health and social care professions involves the continual acquisition, review and application of different types of explicit and tacit knowledge derived from different information sources (Eraut 1994), which collectively underpin judgements, decisions and interventions. Four types of knowledge are identified as encoded, embodied, embrained and embedded (Lam 2000):

- **Encoded knowledge** – Theory, research, applied physical and social sciences, professional code, policies, standardized procedures (Chapter 1), clinical guidelines, legislation.
- **Embodied knowledge** – Personal understanding, sensory, psychomotor (practical), affective (emotional) and interpersonal skills associated with experience and intuition (Chapter 1).
- **Embrained knowledge** – Capacity to process and evaluate information, systematic problem solving, reflection (Chapter 1), critical and creative thinking skills (Chapter 2/3).
- **Embedded knowledge** – Contextual, cultural, collaborative understanding of social/political system (Chapter 2/3), local customs, values, shared routines and working practices.

Encoded knowledge is explicit, in the public domain (published work), and its claims, principles, rationale and supporting evidence are open to scrutiny by others. It is referred to as 'espoused theory' (Argyris 1992) when used by practitioners to explain or justify decisions and actions but there may be other, sometimes more significant influencing factors, which are difficult to articulate. Embodied (personal) and embedded (cultural) knowledge are mainly tacit as they occur below individual or group consciousness and so remain largely unnoticed. They may be referred to as 'theories-in-use' (Argyris 1992) including practitioners' perceptions, attitudes, or taken for granted assumptions which can drive behaviour but are hard to identify or explain.

Embrained knowledge is also tacit when used to intuitively process embodied or embedded knowledge but it becomes more explicit through post-graduate education and when used to analyse encoded knowledge.

Where knowledge and understanding derived from explicit, encoded, espoused theory do not match that derived from tacit, embodied/embedded theories-in-use, a theory–practice gap occurs, for example, antiseptic hand-scrub is placed in a clinical area to clean hands between each patient contact in order to combat cross-infection but it is rarely used. A theory-gap can possibly be reduced where the relevance of theory can be demonstrated by applying it to enhance professional practice, for example, health promotion to limit alcohol consumption to safe levels and the consequences of not doing so (alcohol-related disease, accidents and anti-social behaviour). A theory–practice gap could also be reduced by making tacit embodied/embedded knowledge more visible to develop relevant theory, for example, qualitative research exploring nurses' perceptions and experiences of clinical decision-making led to the creation of a matrix model (Chapter 1).

Clinical governance and risk management

The current shift in emphasis from clinical autonomy to clinical governance in health and social care is associated with valuing encoded knowledge over embodied or embedded knowledge. One of the key issues behind this movement is how to interpret risk: as a hazard that can lead to blame and litigation from which practitioners and organizations should be protected (risk avoidance) or as a way for empowering users (risk taking). The climate is more oriented towards the former rather than the latter and the educational implication of this is that learning more explicit technical skills in formal settings is regarded as the best way to equip and protect employers and professionals. The judgement and decision-making processes of individual practitioners and organizations' protocols are under greater scrutiny, particularly in relation to risk management. These external pressures are leading health and social care practitioners, professional bodies, and educators to affirm 'our decision-making must become more focused, accurate and accountable' (Taylor 2006: 1201). Encoded knowledge is more easily identified and explained in justifying judgements and decisions.

The inherent unpredictability and uncertainty of health and social care require advanced practitioners to be able to take calculated risks as well as manage known risks (Chapter 2). Sometimes statistical evidence enables identification of certain risk categories, for example, morbidity and mortality rates associated with diet, exercise and lifestyle. At other times, for example, assessing whether a child is in danger of being abused, judgement is also informed by embodied and embedded knowledge when interacting with families in their own homes and with relevant agencies. Research has demonstrated that tacit knowledge or 'gut feeling' can represent a multilayered mix of cognitive abilities and activities (embrained knowledge) including focusing, problem solving, thinking laterally and holistically, and ability to work smarter (Gerber 2001: 79). Hence, encoded, embodied, embrained and embedded knowledge are all valuable to practitioners and need various types of lifelong learning or professional development activities to enhance them.

Models of lifelong learning in professional practice

The road to acquire a full range of professional competencies is long and takes place mainly through work-based learning in clinical practice. In order to negotiate the journey of professionalization from initial qualification to advanced levels of expertise many 'maps' (ways of learning) are available. Models of lifelong learning, in acquiring different types of knowledge underpinning judgement and decision-making, come from opposing philosophical traditions. A positivist philosophy of knowledge (epistemology) underpins the physical sciences, establishes cause and effect relationships, and applies universal laws. 'Technical rationality' is a model of learning associated with this scientific tradition which has been influential in medicine and the allied health professions. An interpretive tradition underpins phenomenology (Chapter 1) and symbolic interaction, where meaningful knowledge is thought to be socially constructed as people interact within their environments. 'Knowing-in-action', 'community of practice', 'knowing-in-practice', and 'expansive learning' are models of learning associated with phenomenological and interactionist traditions of human inquiry.

Technical rationality

Technical rationality (Schön 1983) refers to the adoption of rigorous scientific methods to control bias in generating reliable, objective, quantifiable facts to explain, predict or manipulate changes in the environment. In this approach professional knowledge is explicit, encoded and embrained, involving the application of scientific evidence and techniques to resolve human problems in health and social care. For example, understanding drug doses, the physiological effect of medicines, the physical conditions they are intended to treat and the potential unwanted side effects to watch out for involve applying technical rationality.

Knowing-in-action

Knowing-in-action (Schön 1983) assumes that competent practitioners usually know more than they can say. They know how to do their work but not how to describe it. Evidence of such tacit, embodied knowledge is obtained by observing practitioners in their daily work. Knowing-in-action also involves applying embrained knowledge to selectively manage a large amount of information, looking at several things at once without disrupting the flow of inquiry, and making inferences. In other words it is the ability to keep in mind, and work simultaneously on, a variety of data and processes related to each other but forming independent strands. A decision results from a series of parallel creative lines of inquiry that is neither entirely linear nor explicit. Knowing-in-action is a spiral of appreciation, action, and re-appreciation. Understanding through the attempt to change, and changing through the attempt to understand is the distinctive nature of knowing-in-action. For example, facilitating group work enabling clients to both give and receive psychotherapeutic support involves applying knowing-in-action.

Community of practice

In a community of practice (Wenger 1998) learning occurs through engaging and participating in group or collective life. Such participation is called a community of practice. Learning is seen as a social process taking place when people who have common goals interact as they strive towards achieving them. It is based on the original work of anthropologists Barbara Rogoff and Jean Lave who explored how learning occurred in apprenticeship settings. The term 'community of practice' described communities of practitioners into which newcomers would enter in order to acquire knowledge and skills embedded in the crafts and practices of the community. Such learning is acquired through legitimate peripheral participation (Wenger 1998). Legitimate, meaning people need to be accepted in order to join a community of practice. Peripheral, meaning new members are allowed to practise simple or low-risk tasks that are nevertheless productive. Participation, meaning members gradually take part in all aspects of the community of practice. This includes its tasks, unique vocabulary, and organizing principles so that they may become expert practitioners. The process of legitimate peripheral participation in a community of practice appears to complement a novice to expert transition in the skill acquisition model (Dreyfus and Dreyfus 1986).

Knowing-in-practice

In knowing-in-practice (Gherardi et al. 2003) lifelong learning is situated, meaning it has to be understood in relation to the specific characteristics of the clinical context where it is generated and applied. Hence, it is socially constructed embodied and embedded professional knowledge and cannot be reduced to component parts, decontextualized or abstractly represented and transmitted from one person to another. For example, starting a new job is unsettling until local customs and practices are understood. The final state of organized work cannot be predicted in advance but unfolds over time and activities. The functions of setting up, organizing, co-ordinating and running processes are distributed over a variety of roles and responsibilities.

Knowing-in-practice combines and complements elements of knowing-in-action and community of practice models but also suggests how unpredictable events offer unique, learning opportunities by 'stretching' practitioners' coping skills (Cheetham and Chivers 2001) to make on the spot decisions. Legitimate peripheral participation in a community of practice does not account for learning prompted by 'stretching' experiences where practitioners' repertoire of judgement and decision-making skills are insufficient to cope with stresses and challenges of unforeseen circumstances. Such experiences lie at the boundaries of practitioners' comfort zone involving 'touching the limits of what is known'. They occur when practitioners are exposed to situations where routine judgement and decision-making are suspended and ad hoc processes have to be initiated but may only be possible in a 'blame-free' culture. For example, Chapter 1 described critical incidents where newly registered nurses coped with emergency situations including reviving a baby who had stopped breathing, despite never having done so before and being the only nurse present. Organizations may also experience 'stretching' when systems fail to manage a discrepancy between supply and demand for services. This can trigger 'double loop learning' by questioning and revising assumptions, values, existing policies, systems or strategies, to adapt to changing circumstances (Argyris 1992). This might involve increasing staffing levels in the above example.

Expansive learning

Expansive learning (Engeström 2001) is the most complex form of lifelong learning because it combines elements of all the other models and types of knowledge, it does not separate individual from organizational learning, and it focuses on continuous transformation to face new challenges. In this sense it contributes to ongoing radical exploration and reconfiguration of complex adaptive 'whole systems' (Chapter 3), encouraging collaboration between all stakeholders (subsystems) to identify, implement and coordinate creative solutions as social change presents new challenges.

Expansive learning is derived from activity theory (associated with Soviet psychologist, Vygotsky) which assumes that when individuals engage and interact with their environment, they produce tools (cultural artefacts) such as documents. These tools are manifestations of mental processes which then become more accessible and communicable to other people through social interaction.

Activity theory is based on five principles:

1. Activity system as the unit of analysis: Activity system analysed in its network relations to other activity systems. For example, a form assessing a child's needs, used in a social care team, is used to inform a multi-agency plan of action regarding the child. It is only through starting from one system that we can make sense of the entire network or whole systems. Activity systems realize and reproduce themselves by generating agreed plans and actions.

2. Multi-voiceness of activity: An activity system is always part of a wider community of multiple points of view, traditions or interests and so collaboration of all relevant parties is essential.
3. Historicity of activity: Activity systems take shape and get transformed over lengthy periods of time. Their problems and potentials are only understood in relation to their own history.
4. Contradictions as a driving force of change in activity: Contradictions are historically accumulating structural tensions within, and between, activity systems. For example, the tension between individual and social responsibility to meet health and social care needs.
5. Expansive cycle as a possible form of transformation in activity: Activity systems move through relatively long cycles of qualitative transformations. As the contradictions of an activity system are aggravated, established norms are questioned and this prompts change. For example, emergency care is recognized as a priority 24-hour service but some important support services are only available from 9 am–5 pm Monday to Friday. In Chapter 1 this contributed to the death of a patient with a head injury, the severity of which was not detected as no radiologist was available to conduct a cranial CT scan. It would, therefore, appear necessary for important support services to be available 24 hours.

Informal work-based lifelong learning strategies

Practitioners and professionals learn through formal learning both at the beginning (the course and programme leading to their qualification) and throughout (from professional development programmes, both sponsored by their employers and self-funded) their career. However, research demonstrates that learning achieved through informal experiences is equally relevant for achieving full competency as felt by the professional concerned and by his/her colleagues (Cheetham and Chivers 2001). Thus formal and informal learning are inter-related processes with the latter appearing to be more significant over time. On the job learning was considered the most important informal learning process, followed by working alongside more experienced colleagues, and working as part of a team. It seems that professionals value all those informal learning activities associated with practising and performing their professional role, being supported by colleagues, and having shared goals. Therefore, in social care and healthcare, professional practice is not just doing but also learning from doing and building upon existing mental models derived from previous experience. This is what Schön (1983) refers to as repertoires of solutions.

Repertoires of solutions can be developed with reference to a classification (taxonomy) of twelve informal work-based learning methods ranging from simple to more complex activities (Cheetham and Chivers 2001). They were developed from research including a literature review, surveying a wide range of professional occupations (including health), and interviewing respondents to find out what helped them acquire, develop and apply the knowledge and skills needed for their practice while they were at work.

The 'PROFESSIONAL' taxonomy of informal work-based learning (Cheetham and Chivers 2001: 281), including some examples, is described below:

P   Practice and repetition: simulations, emergency drill, rehearse/perform procedures

R   Reflection: individual and/or group reflection 'in' (present) and 'on' (past) practice

O   Observing and copying: shadow positive role models as a benchmark to emulate

F   Feedback: positive and negative criticism from colleagues, managers, service users

E   Extra-occupational transfer: previous jobs/life experience/hobbies/interests inform role

S   Stretching activities: act up in a senior role, deal with emergency, pioneer new service

S   Switching perspectives: exchange visits, job swap, experience as a patient, new insights

I   Interaction with coach: mentoring, supervision, sounding board activities, and tutorials

O   Osmosis – unconscious absorption: gain tacit embodied/embedded knowledge via senses

N   Neurological/psychological devices/techniques: problem solving or creative thinking tools

A   Articulation: writing papers, speaking at conferences, and developing learning material

L   Liaison/collaboration: with peers, interprofessional, local/national/international joint projects

Given the practice-based nature of health and social care there are infinite opportunities for work-based learning experiences and the 'PROFESSIONAL' taxonomy offers a useful framework to understand the mechanisms by which practitioners' clinical judgement/decision-making skills can be enhanced. It appears quite comprehensive in embracing tacit and explicit knowledge and phenomenological/interactionist and scientific learning styles referred to previously, for example:

- Osmosis: incorporates embodied and embedded knowledge that practitioners are often unaware of unless a critical incident causes them to consciously reflect upon their practice.
- Stretching activities: stimulate embrained knowledge to find creative solutions to problems.
- Articulation: involves communicating theoretical, encoded knowledge and may also convert hitherto tacit professional knowledge and skills into an explicit narrative that can be shared.
- Neurological/psychological devices: using technical rationality to enhance judgement.

- Practice and repetition: knowing-in-action, skills have to be practised not just demonstrated.
- Interaction with coach: support from an experienced colleague in a community of practice.
- Reflection: unlock mystery of events, examine and reveal details of knowing in practice.
- Switching perspectives: gain insight into other stakeholders' views via expansive learning.

The relevance of the 'PROFESSIONAL' taxonomy in encompassing and facilitating development of a comprehensive range of knowledge and skills in practice settings suggests it could be adopted as a template to establish an effective clinical learning environment in health and social care. It supports established methods, such as mentoring students during practice placements, and clinical supervision to develop registered practitioners clinical judgement and decision-making expertise.

Mentoring and supervision

Many of the work-based learning methods identified by Cheetham and Chivers (2001) can be applied within a 'SCaRCE' mentoring model (Figure 4.1, Standing 1998) developed by critiquing and adapting 'A Comprehensive Mentoring Model' (Anderson and Shannon 1995) for use in nurse education.

The 'SCaRCE' mentoring model complements the 'PROFESSIONAL' taxonomy when experienced nurses are both supportive and challenging in stretching/testing students in practice placements. It also promotes and assesses the development of both thinking (reflective) and practical skills (competency)

MENTORING DISPOSITIONS	MENTORING FUNCTIONS
Openness: Approachable	**Teach**: Transmit professional knowledge and skills
Expressing care/concern: Humane	**Counsel**: Discuss learning options and give advice
Awareness of mentee: Student-centred	
Awareness of political economy of mentoring: Accept responsibility as 'gatekeeper' to protect public	**Support**: Value and help student to manage anxiety
	Reflect: Facilitate self-awareness/critical reflection
	Challenge: Stretch student's knowledge and skills
MENTORING RELATIONSHIPS	MENTORING ACTIVITIES
Role model: Attention on mentor's performance	**Tutorials**: Demonstration of procedures
Nurturer: Maintaining trust and rapport	**Meetings**: Reflect on experience, plan activities
Supervisor: Attention on student's performance	**Observation**: Feedback and assessment of student

Figure 4.1 Supportive/Challenging and Reflective/Competency Education (SCaRCE) mentoring model (Standing 1998)

necessary for effective clinical judgement/decision-making as a registered nurse.

Mentoring is linked to students' pre-registration education and supervision is linked to practitioners' potential lifelong learning in professional practice. Supervision involves applying most of the dispositions, roles, functions and activities associated with mentoring, except that the status of supervisor and supervisee is more equal, as both are registered practitioners. Recognizing the value of and accepting the need for clinical supervision can be a challenge that requires:

> Valuing yourself enough as a practitioner to be able to stop and critically reflect on your practice, with others who are very likely to have similar concerns. This may well mean looking at existing methods of work and making a conscious decision to change them. In order to care for others, it is important that individual practitioners look after themselves, otherwise they will find themselves too much in need of support to be able to give any.
>
> (Driscoll 2000: 195)

Hence, supervision also complements a 'PROFESSIONAL' taxonomy (Cheetham and Chivers 2001) particularly regarding [R] Reflection, [F] Feedback, [S] Switching perspectives, [I] Interactive coach and [L] Liaison/collaboration. Proctor's (1986) interactive model of supervision has three functions:

1. **Restorative/supportive**: Emotional support to cope with work related stresses
2. **Formative/educational**: Reflection and development of knowledge and skills
3. **Normative/managerial:** Monitor effectiveness and quality of clinical practice.

Combining Proctor's three functions through interactive peer supervision helps to review and renew practitioners' affective, cognitive and psychomotor skills, facilitate safe and effective clinical judgement/decision-making and interventions, and foster a positive transformation of practice. The review of practitioners' knowledge and skills in supervision depends on a commitment to reflecting on practice, achieving meaningful learning, and applying this to future practice. This process is summarized in Driscoll's (2000) revised WHAT? Model of structured reflection, as follows:

- **WHAT? (Describe event)**   Describe events from practice with trusted colleague
- **SO WHAT? (Analyse event)**   Obtain feedback and write down what has been learnt
- **NOW WHAT? (Proposed action)**   Take action to apply learning in professional practice

Clinical supervision, therefore, supports lifelong learning and reflective practice in reviewing and developing professional identity and expertise. It also supports clinical governance by monitoring and enhancing the quality and effectiveness of practitioners' judgements, decisions and actions, and it is associated with descriptors of advanced practitioners' leadership skills (Chapter 2).

Reflective activity 4.1

To help you relate theory/research about work/practice-based learning to your own experience:

1. List the twelve methods of informal work-based learning identified in the 'PROFESSIONAL' taxonomy (Cheetham and Chivers 2001) discussed earlier.
2. Look at the examples given for each category, reflect, and relate them to your experience.
3. Write down an example for each of the twelve informal work-based learning methods from your experience that has helped you to develop clinical judgement/decision-making skills.
4. Ask one or two work colleagues to work through above steps (1–3) and arrange to meet up.
5. Compare examples and discuss how to apply the 'PROFESSIONAL' taxonomy to enhance the development of clinical judgement/decision-making skills in your practice area.

Formal learning in continuing professional development programmes

Continuing professional development (CPD) programmes to enhance clinical judgement and decision-making are usually found in higher education institutions. The advantage of CPD is that practitioners have time to reflect on practice, learn about new theoretical perspectives or research, and develop their critical thinking skills. The disadvantages are that they are removed from the clinical context where their knowledge and skills are embedded which can be disempowering for experienced practitioners or clinical managers. This is compounded where there is a perception that higher education involves passively listening to lectures to acquire the explicit, encoded knowledge needed to pass assignments. The removal from practice and temporary displacement within a university can conspire to make mature students feel deskilled and possibly experience a sense of regression, like 'going back to school', associated with a high dependence on lecturers for support. It is, therefore, necessary to dispel rather than perpetuate the impression of such a split between a world of theory and a world of practice and the following strategies can be used to achieve this.

Applying adult learning principles

Judgement and decision-making, taught as part of an MSc Interprofessional Health and Social Care, apply principles of adult learning (andragogy) to empower practitioners to fully participate in their roles as students (Knowles 1980). This assumes that adult learners are:

- Autonomous individuals capable of self-directed learning
- Aware of their learning needs and motivated to address them
- Interested in applying learning to address practical problems
- A rich learning resource of personal and professional experience
- Partners in a collaborative generation and exchange of ideas.

In order to fully engage practitioners and utilize their experience of judgement and decision-making, learning and teaching methods encourage active participation rather than passive listening. In many ways this reflects similar values to those of a work-based learning perspective in recognizing the dynamic nature of learning which can occur incidentally, accidentally, as well as intentionally (Cheetham and Chivers 2001). This approach encompasses the Learning Process Perspective (De Jong 1997) acknowledging students' self-directed learning potential, and the interpretative paradigm (Carr and Kemmis 1983) where learning is an interactive process in which students ascribe meaning to their work-based experience, and it is self-reflective (Mezirow 1985), as students are encouraged to develop self-knowledge and achieve personal goals.

Creating an interprofessional learning community

The emphasis upon students'/practitioners' personal and professional experience and perceptions, while important in making learning sessions productive and relevant, can also be anxiety-provoking particularly if discussing mistakes that occurred in practice. It is, therefore, necessary to ensure the classroom is perceived to be a safe, confidential and supportive holding space otherwise there will be an understandable reluctance to share information. This involves combining elements of a community of practice (Wenger 1998) and expansive learning (Engeström 2001) within a university-based learning community. A learning community is a group of people who are actively engaged in learning from each other (lecturers learn and teach/students teach and learn) as equal partners. They share experiences of practice, commitment to learning and an active involvement in achieving goals. This approach is a useful template for interprofessional programmes enabling 'liaison/ collaboration' and 'switching perspectives' regarded as valuable tools in learning from other disciplines (Cheetham and Chivers 2001). In effect, the classroom mirrors a 'whole system' of health and social care professionals (nurses, radiographers, physiotherapists, social workers, occupational therapists) reflecting upon and exploring the situated nature of clinical judgement and decision-making in their professional practice. Adopting a learning community approach takes practitioners' clinical experience as a starting point for discussion and enables their respective contributions to health and social care to be shared, examined and valued. It also highlights any current issues, problems and tensions in clinical practice as a basis for considering alternative perspectives in finding a solution and developing new strategies and interventions to effect change.

Theoretical perspectives of judgement and decision-making theory are not taught in isolation but related to students' recollection and identification of issues affecting their practice. This helps to ensure that connections are made linking relevant theory to practice. For example, cognitive continuum theory (Standing 2008) is presented in a workshop format involving students identifying different types of clinical decisions from their practice, what informs them, how they are made, and reviewing alternative options in matching intuitive versus analytic decisions to problems.

Experiential learning

The participative nature of such workshops encourages students to actively engage in new learning experiences, reflect on how they relate to practice, consider new frameworks to help guide or explain judgements, and then test them out to see if they can be applied to enhance practice. This reflects a cycle of experiential learning (Kolb 1984; Honey and Mumford 1986) as follows:

- Concrete experience
- Observation and reflection
- Abstract conceptualization and generalization
- Active experimentation and testing out ideas.

Grounding learning in experiential activities helps to offset some of the disadvantages of being removed from the clinical context in which judgement is usually exercised. It also enables informal as well as formal learning to occur and stimulates awareness of tacit knowledge as well as theory. It requires a high commitment from students but rewards are commensurate as their experience is valued, they are not passive recipients of transmitted knowledge but active in discovery learning, and, in the symbolic interactionist tradition they co-create relevant socially constructed knowledge.

It also depends upon students being suitably experienced to reflect and connect theory to practice as 'it may be that reflection does not become fully effective until practitioners have built up sufficient experience against which to reflect' (Cheetham and Chivers 2001: 270). Such experience can lead to 'template modelling' (Boreham 1987) where professionals develop and store mental models from previous experience and apply them to new encounters which may complement or clash with others' views and theoretical perspectives (Schön 1983). It is, therefore, important to devise ways of eliciting and discussing students'/practitioners' tacit knowledge, beliefs, attitudes, values

and skills in relation to their clinical judgement and decision-making responsibilities.

Techniques to engage health professionals in participative learning

Some techniques to help elicit students' knowledge, beliefs, values and experience include questioning and mapping the development of judgement
and decision-making skills are:

- How/Where/When did you originally learn clinical judgement and
  decision-making?
- How/Where/When/What do you do to keep up to date regarding clinical
  judgement?
- Describe any recent experience of clinical decision-making that you were
  involved in.
- What evidence supported the decision, what action resulted, and who else
  contributed?
- How would you like to improve regarding your clinical judgement
  decision-making skills?

This exercise is followed by group discussions situating students' judgement
and decision-making experience within a social, political, economic and professional context, using prompts such as:

**How do you perceive the following influences to impact on your
judgement and decision-making?**

- Your personal/practical/professional knowledge, skills, experience and expectations of self?
- Public/patients/clients/service users/consumers rights, needs, hopes and
  expectations?
- Peers, work colleagues, different health/social care professionals, and other
  agencies?
- Managers/administrators, supervisors, auditors, organizational struc-
  ture/culture/values?
- Standards of practice and code of conduct specified by your professional
  regulatory body?
- Central/local government, social policy, legislation, demographic and economic factors?

Students are then asked to do a force field analysis (Lewin 1943) to plan
a transformation from the present to a future desired state regarding their
judgement/decision-making skills. This involves mapping and assessing contradictory forces that block their energy/creative potential and then making
changes to enable positive forces to outweigh negative ones. It also offers an
opportunity to integrate and apply previously identified influences in students' force field analyses.

Reflective activity 4.2

This activity enables you apply force field analysis in analysing and overcoming obstacles regarding your preferred objectives.

 1. Specify a vision of your future practice regarding the use of advanced judgement/decision-making expertise in a clinical and organizational context that enhances health/social care.
 2. Draw a line down the middle of the page making two columns.
 3. List all the positive driving forces which will help achieving your aim on the left.
 4. List all the negative restraining forces which will hinder achieving your aim on the right.
 5. Rate each force from 1–5 according to your perception of its weakness or strength.
 6. Total up the scores for driving forces versus restraining forces and compare them.
 7. Consider ways of weakening restraining forces and/or strengthening driving forces.
 8. Identify targets that are in your power to achieve which help to effect desired change.
 9. Compare your force field analysis with others in the group and notice similarities and differences within and between different health and social care professionals.
10. Agree strategies and timeframes to achieve targets and give feedback on progress to group.

The above participative and experiential learning and teaching methods demonstrate application of adult learning principles within a collaborative interprofessional learning community. You can use this tool to help integrate theory/practice and maximize the advantages of university education (time devoted to learning, availability of complementary resources) while minimizing disadvantages (removal from clinical context in which practice knowledge is embedded). In doing so you are contrasting tacit and explicit knowledge and phenomenological/interactionist and scientific learning approaches, all are valued in developing students'/practitioners' ability to benefit from any learning opportunities (formal or informal).

Maximizing work-based learning opportunities

Marsick and Watkins (1990) summarized the personal characteristics required by practitioners to maximize work-based learning opportunities as follows:

1. **Pro-activity:** Readiness to take the initiative in situations
2. **Critical reflection:** Reflecting, not just on events but on underlying assumptions

3. **Creativity:** Enabling person to think beyond their normal point of view.

These characteristics are equally important to maximize university-based learning opportunities. The above learning methods, therefore, facilitate greater consistency and coherence (between the rigour of formal university-based and relevance of informal work-based learning) to enhance practitioners' clinical judgement/decision-making skills in providing excellent health/social care.

Maximizing formal learning opportunities

Continuing interprofessional development programmes in clinical judgement and decision-making are more likely to be relevant to practitioners' learning needs and effective where they:

- Enable incidental, accidental informal learning as well as intentional, formal learning
- Understand that learning and its application take place beyond the control of lecturers
- Utilize multiple methods to facilitate active participation in a peer learning community
- Encourage exploitation of practitioners' experiences as potential learning opportunities
- Develop self-directed and collaborative learners committed to transform their practice.

The overall shift is away from encouraging passive 'learners of content' and towards stimulating active 'learning acquirers' (Cheetham and Chivers 2001: 286). This complements the characteristics associated with advanced practitioners (Chapter 2) which are necessary to continually assess and transform (Engeström 2001) professional practice in anticipating and responding to change. Chapter 7, by an advanced practitioner in radiography, is based on her work as a student (on the above MSc Interprofessional Health and Social Care) in developing clinical judgement and decision-making skills further, and applying them to enhance and transform professional practice.

Reflective activity 4.3

The questions that follow are intended to support the achievement of the chapter objectives:

1. Describe the main differences between the way you learned how to reach a judgement or make a decision when you entered your profession compared to how you do it now.

2. In what way have the formal professional development programmes you have attended influenced the development and use of your clinical judgement and decision-making skills?
3. In what way have formal professional development programmes you have attended enabled you/students to contribute/transfer knowledge and skills from practice to sessions?
4. Identify any theories, models or frameworks that you have found helpful in guiding your clinical judgement and decision-making and describe an example of how you applied them.

Chapter summary

This chapter began by sketching the socio-political context which has shaped changes in welfare provision and requires health and social care practitioners to demonstrate effective clinical judgement and decision-making skills. The importance of utilizing and enhancing work-based learning opportunities was emphasized because of their contextual, social and clinical relevance to the development of practitioners' clinical judgement and decision-making skills. This potentially enables relevant tacit/explicit knowledge and ways of learning to be applied to practice and a 'PROFESSIONAL' taxonomy (Cheetham and Chivers 2001) was recommended to facilitate this. Attention then focused on demonstrating how formal university-based programmes can be made more relevant to practice by applying adult/experiential learning principles in an interprofessional peer learning community. This, it is argued, enables transition from passive 'learners of content' to active 'learning acquirers' to support and equip practitioners to transform their clinical practice.

Key points

- Health/social care practitioners need lifelong learning to adapt skills in a changing environment.
- Practitioners' espoused theory refers to explicit/encoded (theoretical) knowledge but everyday theories-in-use usually incorporate tacit/embodied (personal)/embedded (practical) knowledge.
- Practitioners learn embodied/embedded knowledge/skills via legitimate peripheral participation in communities of (healthcare) practice which develop professional knowing-in-action/practice.
- Expansive learning combines individual practitioner and organizational learning in a continuous transformation to face new challenges and adapt practice in dynamic, complex whole systems.
- Invaluable, informal, work-based incidental/accidental learning in healthcare practice is enabled by reflection, role models, mentoring/supervision, 'stretching' activities and using decision tools.

• Formal learning in continuing professional development should promote practitioners' active participation, using their experience as a shared learning resource, to relate theory to practice.

References

Alaszewski, A. (2001) The impact of the Bristol Royal Infirmary disaster and inquiry on public services in the UK. *Journal of Interprofessional Care*, 16: 371–8.

Anderson, E.M. and Shannon, A.L. (1995) Toward a conceptualisation of mentoring, in T. Kerry and A.S. Shelton Mayes (eds) *Issues in Mentoring*. London: Routledge.

Argyris, C. (1992). *On Organizational Learning*. Oxford: Blackwell Publishing.

Boak, G. and Thompson, D. (1998) *Mental Models for Managers*. London: Century Business Books.

Boreham, N.C. (1987) Learning from experience in diagnostic problem solving, in J. Richardson et al. (eds) *Student Learning: Research into education and cognitive psychology*. Guilford: Society for Research into Higher Education, pp. 89–97.

Carr, W. and Kemmis, S. (1983) *Becoming Critical: Knowing through Action Research*. Victoria: Deakin University Press.

Cheetham, G. and Chivers, G. (2001) How professionals learn in practice: an investigation of informal learning amongst people working in professions. *Journal of European Industrial Training*, 25: 246–92.

De Jong, J.A. (1997) Research into on-the-job training: a state of the art. *International Journal of Educational Research*, 25: 449–71.

Dreyfus, H.L. and Dreyfus, S.E. (1986) *Mind over Machine: The power of human intuition expertise in the era of the computer*. Oxford: Basil Blackwell.

Driscoll, J. (2000) *Practising Clinical Supervision: A reflective approach*. Edinburgh: Bailliere Tindall.

Engeström, Y. (2001) Expansive learning at work: towards an activity theoretical reconceptualization. *Journal of Education and Work*, 14: 133–56.

Eraut, M. (1994) *Developing Professional Knowledge and Competence*. London: Falmer Press.

Gerber, R. (2001) The concept of common sense in workplace learning and experience. *Education and Training*, 43: 72–81.

Gherardi, S. and Nicolini, D. (2002) Learning in a constellation of interconnected practice: canon or dissonance? *Journal of Management Studies*, 39: 419–36.

Gherardi, S., Nicolini, D. and Yanow, D. (2003) *Knowing in Organizations: A practice-based approach*. New York: ME Sharpe Publishing.

Honey, P. and Mumford, A. (1986) *The Manual of Learning Styles*. Maidenhead: P. Honey.

Jasper, M. (2003) *Foundations in Nursing and Health Care: Beginning reflective practice*. Cheltenham: Nelson Thornes.

Kemshall, H. (2002) *Risk, Social Policy and Welfare*. Buckingham: Open University Press.

Knowles, M.S. (1980) *The Modern Practice of Adult Education: From pedagogy to andragogy*. New York: Cambridge Books.

Kolb, D.A. (1984) *Experiential Learning*. Englewood Cliffs, NJ: Prentice-Hall.

Lam, A. (2000) Tacit knowledge, organizational learning and societal institutions – an integrated framework. *Organizational Studies*, 21: 487–513.

Lewin, K. (1943) Defining the "Field at a given time". *Psychological Review*, 50: 292–310. Republishing in *Resolving Social Conflicts and Field Theory in Social Science*. Washington, DC: American Psychological Association.

Marsick, V.J. and Watkins, K.E. (1990) *Informal and Incidental Learning in the Workplace.* London: Routledge.

Mezirow, J. (1985) A critical theory of self-directed learning, in S. Brookfield (ed.) *Self-directed Learning: From theory to practice.* San Francisco: Jossey-Bass, pp. 18–22.

Mintzberg, H. (1979) *The Structuring of Organizations: A synthesis of the research.* Englewood Cliffs, NJ: Prentice-Hall.

Proctor, B. (1986) Supervision: a cooperative exercise in accountability, in M. Marken and M. Payne (eds) *Enabling and Ensuring – Supervision in Practice.* Leicester: National Youth Bureau, Council for Education and Training in Youth and Community Work, pp. 21–34.

Purdy, M. (1999) The health of which nation? Health, social regulation and the new consensus, in M. Purdy and D. Banks (eds) *Health and Exclusion.* London: Routledge.

Schön, D.A. (1983) *The Reflective Practitioner: How professionals think in action.* New York: Basic Books.

Standing, M. (1998) Developing a supportive/challenging and reflective/competency education (SCaRCE) mentoring model and discussing its relevance to nurse education. *Mentoring and Tutoring,* 6(3): 3–17.

Standing, M. (2008) Clinical judgement and decision-making in nursing – nine modes of practice in a revised cognitive continuum. *Journal of Advanced Nursing,* 62: 124–34.

Taylor, B.J. (2006) Factorial surveys: using vignettes to study professional judgement. *British Journal of Social Work,* 36: 1187–207.

Wenger, E. (1998) *Communities of Practice, Learning, Meaning and Identity.* Cambridge: Cambridge University Press.

Cognitive continuum theory – nine modes of practice

Mooi Standing

Overview

This chapter describes the key features of contrasting intuitive/experiential and analytic/rational decision theories, discusses their strengths, weaknesses and applications in healthcare, and shows how they are combined in cognitive continuum theory. The main principles of cognitive continuum theory are explained regarding the need to match cognitive tactics to the different demands of decision tasks, and the competences needed to achieve this. Its application to medicine is discussed before critiquing, revising and applying cognitive continuum theory to nursing. Detailed examples and in-depth reflective activities enable readers to relate intuitive/experiential, analytic/rational, and cognitive continuum theories to their own area of clinical practice.

Objectives

- Identify strengths and weaknesses of intuitive/experiential and analytic/rational decisions
- Describe and apply a Lens model of intuitive judgement/decision-making to healthcare
- Describe and apply Bayes' theorem of analytic judgement/decision-making to healthcare
- Understand how the cognitive continuum combines intuitive and analytic decision theories
- Describe and apply cognitive continuum theory (with six modes of inquiry) to medicine
- Describe and apply cognitive continuum theory (with nine modes of practice) to nursing

Contrasting intuitive/experiential and analytic/rational decision theories

Decision theory is linked to the development of social and cognitive psychology and research into perception, information processing, judgement, decision-making, and social behaviour. Two rival theories are:

- **Intuitive/experiential** – associated with evolutionary and social learning of human judgement as part of everyday life to adapt to environmental and social change (Brunswik 1943); and
- **Analytic/rational** – associated with formal education in science, mathematics, statistics to increase the accuracy of decisions in scientifically controlled environments (Edwards 1954).

They are also known as 'System 1' and 'System 2' decision theories (Kahneman et al. 1982). Cognitive continuum theory (Hammond 1978, 1996) combines intuitive/experiential and analytic/rational theories within a single framework matching different decision-making tactics to the varied demands of decision tasks. The main features of the two approaches are contrasted in Table 5.1.

Table 5.1 Intuitive/experiential versus analytic/rational decision theory

Features	Intuitive/experiential (system 1)	Analytic/rational (system 2)
Key people	Brunswik 1943, 1956; Heider 1944, 1958; Hammond 1955; Gigerenzer 1991	Edwards 1954; Savage 1954; Simon 1957; Kahneman, Slovic and Tversky 1982
Theory type	**Descriptive**: observe and describe how people attend to and interpret information cues in natural settings/social contexts to inform their judgement/decisions/actions	**Normative and prescriptive**: statistical probabilities calculated from database frequencies to inform rational decision-making and systematic problem solving.
Associated metaphor	**Lens**: reality perceived through lens that consists of many observable information cues that are used to draw inferences re. underlying conditions or characteristics	**Gambler**: applying the laws of chance to distinguish between favourable and unfavourable odds and predicting the likelihood of different events occurring
Main principles	Judgement is the product of interaction between individual and environment and cannot be understood by studying either in isolation. Humans are goal directed but surrounded by uncertainty and perception is fallible so use range of information cues to make sense of social contexts and **'weigh up' best option** in decisions	Human judgement is unreliable due to bias. Experimental research best way to minimize bias: identify independent and dependent variables; hypothesize/ test cause/effect relationship in controlled laboratory setting; results analysed using **statistical probabilities** of their predictive value and margins of error
Knowledge type	**Tacit**: embodied and embedded content-intuitive embrained process	**Explicit**: encoded content – analytic embrained process
Evaluation of competence	**Correspondence competence**: accurate observation, relevant, practical outcome	**Coherence competence**: consistent, retraceable, rigorous, logical process

(continued)

Table 5.1 Intuitive/experiential versus analytic/rational decision theory (*Continued*)

Features	Intuitive/experiential (system 1)	Analytic/rational (system 2)
Related theory and research	**Lens model**, Social judgement/attribution theory; Observation in natural settings	Decision analysis tools – **Bayes' theorem**, Prospect theory, Laboratory experiment
Test of validity in re-searching decision-making	**Ecological validity** Internal: Identified cues truly represent uncertain situation inferences relate to External: Sample representative of social context to which results generalized	**Scientific validity** Internal: Random selection/ allocation to double blind experimental/control group External: Sample representative of wider population to which results generalized
Strengths	**Relevance**: portrays dynamic complexity of everyday human judgement as people interact within their local social contexts	**Rigour**: generate scientific knowledge via research that is open to scrutiny and can be replicated to minimize bias/error
Weaknesses	Local focus may **ignore topical, national studies**. Human perception, information processing and judgement prone to error	Laboratory experiments can be artificial/**unrepresentative of social contexts** or their influence on individual judgement
Applications in healthcare	Professional 'knowing-in-action/ practice', **reflective practice**, patient-centred care	'Technical rationality', **evidence-based practice**, systematic nursing process

Table 5.1 outlines how each approach to decision theory has different strengths, weaknesses and applications to clinical judgement and decision-making in nursing/interprofessional healthcare, and we explore these below.

Intuitive/experiential decision theory

This explains how tacit, embodied/embedded knowledge and 'knowing-in-action/practice', gained through informal work-based/social learning (Chapter 4), enables interpretation of observations to inform judgement and decision-making. For example, Benner's (1984) account of expert nurses' intuitive judgement and Schön's (1987) reflection-in/on-action in professional practice. Similarly, 'Experience and intuition', 'Observation' and 'Reflective' perceptions of clinical decision-making skills, identified in the matrix model (Chapter 1), also indicate application of intuition and experience.

Practitioners' competence is demonstrated where outcomes of decisions have a direct practical benefit. This requires accurate observation and understanding of relevant information cues which contribute to effective assessment, responsive problem solving, and judgement/decision-making that addresses the unique demands of a clinical context. Collectively, these skills are referred to as correspondence competence (Hammond 1996), as decisions and actions need to correspond to the practical realities of decision tasks. Tacit knowledge and intuitive judgement are subconscious processes making it difficult to clearly explain the reasons for decisions. This puts more emphasis on whether a patient/client benefits from an intervention to justify clinical decisions. If the outcome is poor, correspondence competence is seen to be lacking, and it is difficult to defend decisions.

The tacit nature of intuitive/experiential decision-making and 'knowing-in-action/practice' suggests there may be a considerable body of knowledge in nursing and interprofessional healthcare which, although used every day, remains largely invisible because it is not articulated. If this tacit expertise is beneficial to patients/clients, it needs to be developed and protected but, in a culture of evidence-based healthcare, it is under threat unless its effectiveness can be explained and demonstrated. The Lens model (Brunswik 1943, 1956; Heider 1944; Hammond 1955) offers a structure that can be used to understand and explain how subconscious mental processes of tacit knowledge and intuitive judgement inform clinical decisions. Figure 5.1 shows how the Lens model can be applied to illustrate and articulate intuitive judgement/decision-making expertise in a healthcare context.

UNCERTAIN SITUATION	CUE VALIDITY (ECOLOGICAL)	INFORMATION CUES	CUE UTILITY (WEIGHTING)	JUDGEMENT/ DECISION
	←	Stifled crying out	→	
	←	Collapsing	→	
	←	Grimacing	→	
Patient's sudden deterioration in health status	←	Unable to move	→	Heart attack
	←	Pallor	→	Call 'crash' team
	←	Sweating	→	Stabilize heart
	←	Difficulty breathing	→	
	←	Severe chest pain	→	
⇧	←	Pain going down arm	→	⇩
	←	Indigestion	→	
	←	Radial pulse not recordable	→	

⇐ OUTCOME OF DECISION **(CORRESPONDENCE COMPETENCE)** ⇐

Figure 5.1 Lens model: intuitive judgement/decision-making in a healthcare situation

The Lens model is so called because the identified information cues act like a lens through which the uncertain nature of reality is perceived (Hammond 1996). Which cues practitioners choose to attend to, judge to be stronger indicators than others, and how they apply this information to make decisions is guided by experience and rules of thumb (heuristics). For example, individually the information cues (Figure 5.1) are signs/symptoms of many medical conditions but collectively they support the provisional diagnosis of a heart attack which prompts urgent investigation and action. Information is perceived through the senses, for example, the cues in Figure 5.1 involve sight, sound and touch. Some cues warrant higher weighting than others in conveying clues about underlying conditions, for example, chest pain, difficulty breathing and pain going down the arm are stronger indicators of a heart attack than crying out, grimacing and being unable to move. Some cues only become apparent if the practitioner investigates further, for example, asking a patient where it hurts or recording vital signs. The practitioner's judgement/decision-making skill involves observing and recognizing the significance of information cues (signs/symptoms) and applying this to select appropriate interventions that address problems. The Lens model can be used to analyse, evaluate and develop judgement/decision-making skills in learning to attend to relevant information cues, understanding their relative strength/weighting as indicators of health problems (ecological validity/ cue utility), and taking action to effect a positive outcome (correspondence competence). It can, therefore, complement evidence-based practice by articulating practitioners' tacit, experiential skills.

The Lens model has inspired research into how people are able to exercise reasonably accurate judgement in adapting to their social contexts. Brunswik (1943, 1956) pioneered 'representative design' arguing that psychological research must take place in (represent) social contexts where judgement/decision-making usually occurs rather than the artificial setting of a research laboratory. Brunswik advocated use of situation sampling, involving observing and testing how an individual uses judgement in a range of tasks within their social context, rather than population sampling where a large number of people are asked their opinion about specific issues. For example, he studied one student's ability to judge the height and distance of surrounding buildings or objects in 174 different instances as he accompanied the student walking around a university campus. The student had no measurement aids so relied on visual/spatial cues to inform judgement. Brunswik reported that the student's estimates were consistently close to true, objectively measured values. The relative accuracy of the student's unaided estimates supports the Lens model in explaining how intuitive/experiential judgement/decision-making applies tacit knowledge and skills. The Lens model also influenced the development of attribution theory regarding the weighting given to dispositional (individual) versus situational (environmental) cues when interpreting behaviour (Heider 1958); and social judgement theory applied to social policy, engineering, finance, weather forecasting, legal, and clinical settings (Brehmer and Joyce 1988; Cooksey 1996; Hammond 1996). The Lens model could also be applied to research decision-making in nursing/interprofessional healthcare.

Reflective activity 5.1

This activity is intended to help you understand the Lens model by applying it to reflect on and explore an example from your own experience of clinical judgement/decision-making.

1. Refer to Figure 5.1 'Lens model: intuitive judgement/decision-making in a healthcare situation' and write down the main headings on an A4 sheet of paper.
2. Think about your own recent clinical experience, identify an example where you had to come to a decision, and briefly describe the focus of this under the heading 'Uncertain situation'.
3. Describe the different sources of information that were available to you at the time including all the sensory stimuli you perceived when assessing the patient/client, relevant prior knowledge and experience that assisted you, feedback from other members of the healthcare team, test results and any relevant documentation. List these under the heading 'Information cues'.
4. Reflect upon the value of each cue in conveying vital clues about the uncertain situation you were dealing with (cue validity). Which ones would you say are stronger indicators than others? Individually, could the cues be associated with many different health issues? When you combine the information cue, how does this help to reveal more about the uncertain situation? Did you underestimate the importance of any cues? Did you overestimate the importance of any cues? Were there any important sources of information that were *not* available to you? How might this information have helped you to understand the problem if it had been available?
5. Under the heading 'Judgement/decision' briefly describe your assessment of the situation and proposed action. Reflect upon how the identified information cues individually and collectively influenced your clinical judgement/decision-making and interventions (cue utility). How did you think your proposed action was going to address the issues suggested by the information cues? What alternative decision/action might you have taken and why did you choose not to?
6. Under the heading 'Outcome of decision' describe what happened in relation to the uncertain situation/healthcare problem you were dealing with. Was there any noticeable change in the situation? How do you know whether this resulted from your actions or some other reason? Did the patient/client's response support your initial assessment or did new information cues point to a different provisional diagnosis and/or problem identification? With hindsight, what might you have done differently to achieve a more effective outcome?
7. Reflect upon your application of the Lens model in undertaking this reflective activity. How useful do you find the Lens model in illustrating the structure and function of your own intuitive/experiential judgement and decision-making? How might you apply the Lens model in reflecting upon, explaining and evaluating your clinical judgement and decision-making in the future? What have you learned about your own professional development needs during this activity?

Analytic/rational decision theory

This explains how explicit, encoded/abstract knowledge and 'technical rationality', gained through formal university-based education (Chapter 4) enable the analysis and evaluation of relevant theory, research studies, results of scientific investigations, and quantifiable clinical observations to inform practitioners' judgement and decision-making. This approach is closely associated with the promotion of high quality, accountable, evidence-based practice that applies results from national/international validated scientific research studies to guide and enhance standards of healthcare. Similarly, 'Standardized' and 'Systematic' perceptions of clinical decision-making skills, identified in the matrix model (Chapter 1), also indicate application of analytic and rational decision-making.

Practitioners' competence is demonstrated where the decision-making process used is consistent, logical, retraceable and defensible. This requires the application of critical thinking and systematic problem solving skills to question practice, identify knowledge deficits, search for and evaluate appropriate evidence to address gaps in knowledge, and apply it to inform clinical judgement and decision-making. Collectively, these skills are referred to as coherence competence (Hammond 1996) as decisions require a rigorous, methodical, coherent rationale. Applying explicit scientific and research evidence in analytic/rational decisions is a highly conscious, deliberate process that enables decisions to be scrutinized by others and explained, justified or defended. It emphasizes the value of comparing observations from local clinical practice to national base rates in deciding whether they are within the normal expected range or if further investigation is needed. Morbidity and mortality statistics can also be applied to identify risks and target health promotion.

The coherence and logic of analytic/rational decision theory are associated with understanding and applying statistics to calculate probability values and make informed predictions. Its origins can be traced to Edwards (1954) who studied gambling habits by comparing bets placed with statistical probabilities of winning or losing. The idea that statistics can be used to assist decision-making is central to Prospect theory (Kahneman and Tversky 1979) which describes how potential losses and gains can be evaluated to assess risk. It predicts that people tend to over-react to low probabilities and under-react to high probabilities. For example, it is highly probable that saving money by not buying lottery tickets results in being wealthier than buying lottery tickets in the hope of winning the jackpot (small probability). A recognition that human judgement can result in illogical choices led to the development of decision analysis tools that apply statistics to enable logical, better-informed, more accurate decision-making, for example, Bayes' theorem (Savage 1954; Edwards et al. 1963).

Bayes' theorem can be applied to clinical decisions in risk assessment, diagnosing health problems and predicting outcomes of care on the basis of

Table 5.2 Bayes' theorem: analytic/rational judgement/decision-making in healthcare

Mammography screening of target female population	(A) Assumed incidence of breast cancer in target female population = 1%	(B) Assumed incidence of breast cancer in target Female population = 10%
	Prior Probability	
Number screened	10,000	10,000
Predicted number will test positive for cancer	**100** (1% of 10,000)	**1,000** (10% of 10,000)
Predicted number will test negative for cancer	9,900 (99% of 10,000)	9,000 (90% of 10,000)
	Conditional Probability	
Total testing positive	1,030	1,664
True positive result (sensitivity of test = 80%)	**80** (80% of 100)	**800** (80% of 1,000)
False positive result	**950** (9,900–8,950)	**864** (9,000–8,136)
Total testing negative	8,970	8,336
True negative result (specificity of test = 90.4%)	8,950 (90.4% of 9,900)	8,136 (90.4% of 9,000)
False negative result	20 (100–80)	200 (1,000–800)
	Posterior Probability	
Predictive value of a positive test result	**7.8%** (80 ÷ 1,030 × 100) **(chance of breast cancer)**	**48%** (800 ÷ 1664 × 100) **(chance of breast cancer)**
Predictive value of a negative test result	99.7% (8950 ÷ 8,970 × 100) (chance of *no* breast cancer)	97.6% (8136 ÷ 8,336 × 100) (chance of *no* breast cancer)

known base rates. It can also be used to evaluate the accuracy of scientific evidence and results of investigations including health screening. Table 5.2 shows how Bayes' theorem can be applied to interpret the results of mammography screening.

Just as the Lens model (Figure 5.1) shows how healthcare professionals can manage uncertainty using intuitive/experiential judgement, Bayes' theorem (Table 5.2) shows how uncertainty can be managed using analytic/rational judgement. Both approaches involve making use of available information to reduce uncertainty and inform clinical decisions. The difference between the two lies in the processing of tacit/perceptual versus explicit/statistical knowledge. All aspects of healthcare involve laboratory/technological investigations and tests, so it is important to understand them to evaluate and apply the resulting scientific evidence in the interests of patients/clients. This requires understanding and applying statistical probability, and Bayes' theorem is a useful decision analysis tool in this respect. Table 5.2 identifies three main components in applying Bayes' theorem as:

1. **Determine base rates** – in this case the incidence of female breast cancer (prior probability)
2. **Test and analyse** – separate true and false positive/negative results (conditional probability)
3. **Make an informed prediction** – presence or absence of breast cancer (posterior probability).

These three components of Bayes' theorem can assist practitioners in managing uncertainty, risk assessment and decision-making by comparing local findings with national trends, identifying and adjusting for errors in testing procedures, and establishing the probability of test results being true.

Determine base rates: Just as individual practitioners accumulate experiential knowledge they draw on in facing new situations, national databases continually accumulate facts and figures about the population as a whole that can be used as a reference against which local findings can be compared. Without this wider perspective it is likely that the results of investigative tests such as mammography screening can be misinterpreted. Table 5.2 illustrates this in two examples A and B where the sample size and investigative test are the same but the base rate (assumed incidence of breast cancer) is different (A = 1%, B = 10%). The results are different with 1,030 women testing positive in A as opposed to 1,664 in B. It is not surprising more test positive in B than A as the risk of breast cancer is ten times higher, 10% versus 1%, but it is surprising, given the difference in these base rates, that the results do not show a bigger difference between the two. At this point it is important to compare the numbers predicted to test positive to those actually testing positive. In A only 100 cases are predicted, and yet the results show 1,030 cases. This either means the base rate is wrong and the incidence of breast cancer is higher than 1%, or the test itself is at fault.

Test and analyse: Investigative tests are, themselves, evaluated for quality assurance purposes and as a result their sensitivity (success in detecting a specific condition) and specificity (success in excluding other conditions) rates will be known. It is very unlikely any test will be 100% accurate since all tests are prone to a duality of error in the form of false positive and false negative results (Hammond 1996). Sensitivity for mammography in Table 5.2 is 80%, meaning 80% of women with breast cancer get a true positive result but 20% of women with breast cancer are not detected so get a false negative result (A = 20, B = 200). Specificity for mammography in Table 5.2 is 90.4%, meaning 90.4% of women without breast cancer get a true negative result but 9.6% of women without breast cancer are not excluded so get a false positive result (A = 950, B = 864). It means there are 870 more false than true positive results in A and 64 more false than true positives in B. It is, therefore, essential to recognize and take account of margins of error when interpreting results.

Make an informed prediction: A lack of understanding about the significance of base rates and test sensitivity/specificity rates can lead to results being misinterpreted due to the error of base rate neglect (Kahneman et al. 1982). Intuitively, testing positive for breast cancer is devastating news compounded by the knowledge that the test detects cancer in 80% of cases. Analytically, in order to know the predictive value of tests it is necessary to calculate true positive/negative results as a proportion of the total results. Table 5.2 shows that if the base rate/incidence is 1% of the female population, a positive test result means a 7.8% chance of breast cancer and if the incidence is 10%, a positive test result means a 48% chance of disease. The large number of 'false positives' explain why testing positive for breast cancer means 7.8% risk when the incidence is 1%, mammography sensitivity is 80%, and specificity is 90.4% (Yudkowsky 2003). Screening low risk women appears unsustainable unless mammography specificity is improved. Screening higher risk (incidence 10%) women raises the predictive value of a positive test result six times (48% compared to 7.8%), and more closely reflects a '1 in 9' lifetime risk of female breast cancer (Cancer Research UK 2009).

Bayes' theorem is, therefore, a powerful decision analysis tool requiring basic arithmetic skills to find base rates of a known risk, predict future risk, assess accuracy of risk assessment procedures and effects of inaccuracies, and specify the probability that risk assessment results are true. It can be used to inform clinical judgement/decision-making, managerial decisions, and healthcare policy.

Reflective activity 5.2

This activity is intended to help you understand analytic/rational decision theory by applying Bayes' theorem to analyse testing procedures in your area of clinical practice – a calculator will be helpful.

1. Think about your own area of clinical practice and write down a list of all investigations or tests used to diagnose conditions, risk assessment, or review the effects of treatment interventions.
2. Go through the list and try to identify relevant base rates. This could include the incidence of disease in a given population, normal levels expected in various tests of blood biochemistry, and tests of neurological, physiological and psychological functioning.
3. See if you can identify sensitivity and specificity rates associated with the investigations and tests you identified above. Laboratory test results may indicate what these are but if not, speak to technicians processing the test results and ask them what they are. Relevant research reports evaluating diagnostic tests may also specify sensitivity and specificity rates.
4. Once you have identified both relevant base rates and the sensitivity/specificity of associated tests, this is all the information you need to do

an analysis using Bayes' theorem. Refer to Table 5.2 and draw up your own table – in the left column change the title and the 'predicted number will test positive/negative for?' to suit your example, similarly, change the 'sensitivity/specificity of test' according to rates you identified. In the middle column change the title and specify the relevant base rate/incidence as a percentage. If you wish use to, use third column to specify a much higher base rate/incidence percentage in order to the compare results.

5. Specify sample size e.g. 1,000, calculate predicted number testing positive (multiply sample by your base rate e.g. 1,000 × 2% = 20), calculate predicted number testing negative (multiply sample by 100% minus base rate % e.g. 100% – 2% = 98% × 1,000 = 980). You have now calculated prior probability of the predicted results from the base rate figure you identified.

6. Multiply predicted number testing positive by test sensitivity e.g. 20 × 90% = 18 (true positive), deduct true positive from predicted number testing positive e.g. 20 – 18 = 2 (false negative), multiply predicted number testing negative by test specificity e.g. 980 × 90% = 882 (true negative), deduct true negative from predicted number testing negative e.g. 980 – 882 = 98 (false positive), add true positive to false positive e.g. 18 + 98 = 116 (total testing positive), add true negative to false negative e.g. 882 + 2 = 884 (total testing negative). You have now calculated conditional probability by applying test sensitivity/specificity to predicted results.

7. Divide true positive by total positive and multiply by 100 e.g. 18 ÷ 116 × 100 = 15.5% [chance of positive result being true], divide true negative by total negative and multiply by 100 e.g. 882 ÷ 884 × 100 = 99.7% [chance of negative result being true]. Double check sums. You have now calculated posterior probability by eliminating the effects of false positive/false negative results.

8. Reflect on what you have learned during this activity about: the significance of base rates, the sensitivity and specificity of tests used in your clinical area, the inevitability of false positive and false negative results and their effects on results, use of Bayes' theorem to establish predictive value of positive and negative results, and, value of decision analysis tools to inform decisions.

    •   Did you notice how you had to follow a predetermined, systematic, step-by-step process?
    •   Did you notice how this required you to think logically and use arithmetic skills to analyse results rather than intuition and experience?
    •   Do you understand how easy it can be to misinterpret test results if relying on intuition rather an analytic understanding of what the statistics really mean?
    •   Can you see how explicit and open to scrutiny and challenge your calculations are?
    •   How might you develop and apply your analytic skills further regarding such technological aspects of care?

Combining intuitive/experiential and analytic/rational
in cognitive continuum theory

As summarized in Table 5.1, contrasting intuitive/experiential and analytic/rational decision theories have different strengths, weaknesses and applications. The former is strong on practical relevance and responsiveness but weak on scientific rigour and explanation of judgement/decision-making. The latter is strong on scientific rigour and explanation of judgement/decision-making but weak on practical relevance and responsiveness. Both approaches share an interest in finding the best way to make decisions in facing the ongoing challenge of managing uncertain situations, but they have different ways of achieving this. The intuitive/experiential approach emphasizes participation in the social context and application of tacit knowledge. The analytic/rational approach emphasizes detachment from local contexts and application of explicit knowledge. Hammond (1978) joined the two together in cognitive continuum theory by arguing that different decision tasks require different tactics. He created a system of decision tasks ranging from 'ill structured' to 'well structured' that prompt a response from a system of thinking which ranges from intuition to analysis. The cognitive continuum is, therefore, practice-based and it predicts that more effective decisions and actions result from appropriately matching cognitive tactics to the demands of the situation in question. In this way the intuitive/experiential principle of judgement, being a product of interaction between humans and their environment, is built into the structure of cognitive continuum theory. Similarly, the analytic/rational principle of managing bias and using the most rigorous methods possible according to the nature of decision tasks is also a feature of Cognitive continuum theory. This enables the strengths of both approaches to be combined in a unifying framework that offers a choice of judgement/decision-making tactics to suit variations in the nature of challenges faced. There are five main assumptions of cognitive continuum theory (Hammond 1996):

1. Cognition ranges from intuition to analysis at opposing poles of a continuum. Human reasoning ability is wide-ranging, from spontaneous and intuitive, to logical and analytic.
2. Intuition and analysis are combined (quasirationality) in between the two extremes. Much of the time, judgement/decision-making is not completely intuitive or completely analytic but a bit of both. The proportion of intuition to analysis varies according to the position on the continuum.
3. A continuum of ill/well-structured tasks prompts intuition or analysis or quasirationality. Decision tasks prompting intuition include: managing unexpected or unfamiliar situations or dealing with many issues simultaneously without an existing applicable procedure to guide action. Decision tasks prompting analysis include: managing predictable, controlled situations using a systematic, applicable procedure to guide action. Decision tasks prompting quasirationality combine the two.

4. Cognition is flexible continually moving in either direction along the continuum. Flexibility is needed to be able to continually adjust cognition in response to the different demands and changing nature of decision tasks. Where a chosen tactic is effective there will be no pressure to change but where it is not effective, it will stimulate the search for a more effective alternative.

5. Cognition can recognize general patterns and specific functional relations. Pattern recognition is the ability to collate many information cues at once. Recognizing functional relations is the ability to systematically assess cause and effect relationships between two or more cues. For example, in Chapter 1, a nurse quickly assessed a patient was having a heart attack by simultaneously observing pallor, grimacing, clammy feel to skin, and listening to the patient's description of chest pain (pattern recognition). An electrocardiogram (ECG) machine was then used so the team could monitor any cardiac arrhythmias that might explain the symptoms, and provide a feedback mechanism regarding the patient's response to treatment (functional relations).

Six modes of inquiry along the cognitive continuum (Hammond 1978, 1996)

Hammond subdivided the cognitive continuum into six modes to represent different variations of intuitive and analytic tactics associated with variations in the structure of decision tasks:

1. Physical science experiment:	**pure analysis**	**well structured**
2. Control group experiment:	very strong analysis some intuition	T
3. Quasi-experiment:	strong analysis moderate intuition	A
4. Computer modelling:	strong intuition moderate analysis	S
5. Expert judgement:	very strong intuition some analysis	K
6. Unrestricted judgement:	**pure intuition**	**ill structured**

Hammond's six modes of inquiry show how intuitive/experiential and analytic/rational decision theory are gradually intermingled along the continuum as decision tasks develop a mixture of ill-structured and well-structured elements. The experimental methods of modes 1–3 enable cause and effect functional relations and explicit theoretical knowledge to be tested and procedures are rigorous and transparent, providing an audit trail for others to check or replicate the experiments. Quasi-experiments are the least analytic of these three because they do not use control groups associated with scientific validity and they take place in natural settings, which is more in keeping with representative design, as recommended by Brunswik (1956).

Modes 1–3 are much more painstaking and time-consuming in reaching a conclusion than modes 4–6 where decision-making is quicker, applying tacit knowledge and pattern recognition of simultaneous information cues. Computer modelling is the least intuitive of these three as more time is available to apply decision analysis tools. Choosing the most appropriate mode of inquiry requires accurate assessment and responsiveness to the level of urgency, uncertainty, complexity and structure of decision tasks.

Correspondence and coherence competence in the six modes of inquiry

Whichever mode is being used along the cognitive continuum, the quality of judgement/decision-making can be evaluated with reference to correspondence competence (accurate observation, relevant, practical outcome) and coherence competence (consistent, retraceable, rigorous logical process). As illustrated in Table 5.1, analytic decisions (modes 1–3) are linked to coherence competence but correspondence competence is also needed to match tactics to decision tasks using observation skills. Similarly, intuitive decisions (modes 4–6) are linked to correspondence competence but coherence competence is also needed in the pattern recognition of cues and to explain actions. Hammond (1996) states that correspondence and coherence competence are separate skills, there is no middle ground linking them, so they have to be assessed alternately.

Hamm's application of cognitive continuum theory to medicine

Hamm (1988) recognized the potential of Hammond's cognitive continuum theory as a helpful tool to develop doctors' understanding of clinical judgement and decision-making skills in diagnosing illness and prescribing treatment. Hamm adapted the six modes of inquiry accordingly (Figure 5.2): Modes 1–3 were changed to scientific experiment (in laboratory setting), controlled trial (of new treatment), and quasi-experiment (in health setting). As in Hammond's original framework, more control (possibility of manipulation) and auditability of decisions (visibility of process) occur in modes 1–3 than in modes 4–6, but it increases the time required for interventions. Apart from well-resourced clinical research units, modes 1–3 are less likely to be used than modes 4–6. Modes 4–6 were changed to system-aided, peer-aided, and intuitive judgement. System-aided judgement in medicine ranges from simply 'listing logical possibilities on the back of an envelope' (Dowie 1993: 10) to using decision analysis tools such as Bayes' theorem (Knill-Jones 1993). Peer-aided judgement involves extending professional knowledge by discussing intervention options with experienced colleagues and seeking expert advice where required. Intuitive judgement is the most subjective and private form of cognition involving the use of tacit knowledge, acquired from clinical experience, that doctors are not fully aware of and may be unable to explain.

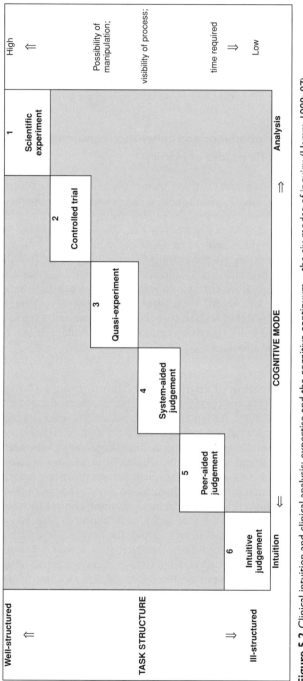

Figure 5.2 Clinical intuition and clinical analysis: expertise and the cognitive continuum – the six modes of inquiry (Hamm 1988: 87)

Dowie (1993) associated a hospital consultant's sequential examination of test results from an in-patient's numerous investigations with applying analytic skills, and a general practitioner's home visit to assess a patient he had not met before with applying intuitive skills. Hamm (1988: 93) noted that doctors mainly use intuitive or peer-aided judgement and recommended they become more analytical using 'appropriate techniques for applying a normative perspective to the case' to help minimize errors. Similarly, Dawes et al. (1989) reported that studies comparing clinicians' intuitive predictions with statistical predictions, derived from the same sources of information, consistently showed the latter to be more accurate. Dowie (1993) advocated doctors using a 'decision tree' (system-aided judgement) to develop analytic skills and improve accuracy in diagnosis and treatment. He used the example of determining whether or not to remove a patient's suspected diseased appendix: plot consequences if the diagnosis is right and if wrong, review outcomes for removing or not removing a diseased or normal appendix with reference to base morbidity and mortality rates, and calculate statistical probabilities regarding identified options.

Using more analytic modes of inquiry does not guarantee mistakes will not be made as findings from experimental research and controlled trials are not infallible. For example, unexpected congenital defects occurred in babies of women prescribed thalidomide for morning sickness while pregnant (Mayers 1977). Hence, errors tend to be 'infrequent but large in the case of analytical tactics, frequent but rarely large in the case of intuition-based tactics' (Hammond 2007: 166). The results of various scientific investigations (biochemistry, haematology, radiology) aiding diagnosis of illness and prescribing treatment are also subject to variations of interpretation: between doctors – 'Inter-observer variability: different clinicians decide upon a different interpretation of the same image or test results'; and by the same doctor – 'Intra-observer variability: the same clinician decides upon a different interpretation of the same image or test result on different occasions' (Muir Gray 1999: 202). This supports the need for continuing education to develop clinicians' use of analytical skills, and, an awareness of the fallibility of information cues and test results in order to enhance the effectiveness and accuracy of clinical decisions and patient safety (Hamm 1988). As discussed earlier, educating health professionals (including doctors) in using Bayes' theorem and other decision analysis tools (system-aided judgement) can help develop the analytic skills necessary to understand relevant statistics and base rates, increase accuracy in interpreting test results, and raise practitioners' awareness of the fallibility of tests (Dowie 1993; Knill-Jones 1993).

Revised cognitive continuum theory – nine modes of practice applied to nursing

The idea of a cognitive continuum ranging from intuition to analysis accommodates nurses who emphasize the value of expert intuitive judgement

(Benner et al. 1996) and those who emphasize the value of evidence-based practice and applying decision analysis tools to reduce decision errors (Lamond and Thompson 2000; Thompson et al. 2004; Harbison 2006). An international survey of nurses' decision-making skills supported the themes of intuition, quasi-rationality and analysis (Lauri et al. 2001). Cognitive continuum theory also accommodates the wide range of descriptive (peer-aided), prescriptive (system-aided) and normative (scientific experiment) decision models (Bell et al. 1995) discussed in Chapter 1. The theory's comprehensiveness is part of its appeal but what makes it especially relevant to nursing/interprofessional healthcare is that it is practice-centred, since the nature of decision tasks determines the type of intervention used.

Just as Hamm (1988) adapted Hammond's cognitive continuum theory for application in medicine (Figure 5.2), Standing (2005, 2008) adapted Hamm's version for application in nursing (Figure 5.3). The revisions include: making it more patient-centred, a broader evidence-base, giving examples of high/low structured nursing tasks, a source of knowledge continuum, an ethical/professional continuum, evaluation criteria for correspondence (effective outcomes) and coherence (logical process) competence, and the six modes of inquiry are replaced by nine modes of practice.

Task structure

The terms 'well' and 'ill' structured tasks, used by Hammond and Hamm, have different meanings in health settings so, to avoid ambiguity, they are replaced by 'high' and 'low'. Examples of high/low structured decision tasks are given reflecting Muir Gray's (1999) distinction between objective/strategic 'faceless' decisions and subjective/operational 'face-to-face' decisions.

Nine modes of practice

As in task structure there is a change of presentation style: the term 'modes of practice' is used instead of 'modes of inquiry' because the inquiry nurses undertake in assessing and addressing patient-centred tasks is an essential part of their professional practice. The nine modes of practice are not numbered because it is not necessary as they are clearly identifiable; and it avoids giving an impression of a preferred hierarchy. The biggest change (Figure 5.3) is to replace six modes of inquiry with nine modes of practice to represent a less restricted, broader evidence base that is more applicable to clinical judgement and decision-making in nursing and interprofessional healthcare. This involves reducing the original six modes to four by combining the three variations of experimental research into one mode, and then adding five new modes: reflective judgement, critical review of experiential and research evidence, action research and clinical audit, qualitative research, and survey research:

- **Intuitive judgement:** forming ideas or opinions without awareness of the process that leads to them (Hammond 1996). For example, insights

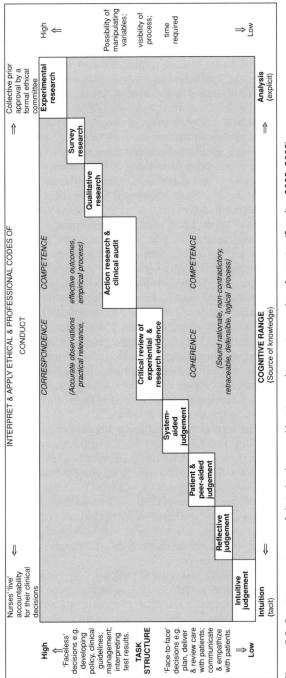

Figure 5.3 Cognitive continuum of clinical judgement/decision-making – nine modes of practice (Standing 2005, 2008)

may occur when a nurse communicates and empathizes with patients, including sensing any changes in their condition that may warrant a more considered risk assessment (Benner and Wrubel 1989). Intuitive judgement is also associated with expert nursing practice including: 'clinical grasp and response-based practice' (recognize and respond to patterns in patients' responses); 'embodied know-how' (combine thinking/knowing/doing to give a fluid, skilled performance); 'seeing the big picture' (wide peripheral vision of clinical context and aware of future possibilities); and 'seeing the unexpected' (salient aspects of situations 'stand out' enabling early detection of problems) (Benner et al. 1996: 45). Chapter 1 indicated that using intuition is not necessarily restricted to expert nurses as some newly registered nurses referred to using it when perceiving and managing critical incidents in clinical practice. However, the subconscious nature of intuition makes it difficult to account for or justify and defend decisions.

- **Reflective judgement:** the ability to consciously, independently think about and reflect upon what you are doing at a given moment (reflection-in-action) and what you have previously experienced (reflection-on-action) (Schön 1987). This important ability is not clearly identified in Hammond's or Hamm's versions of the continuum. Different functions of reflection have been identified in nursing including: reviewing task-related technical competence; communication and interpersonal skills; power relations, advocacy and ethical issues; and dealing with emotions associated with clinical experiences (Johns 2000; Taylor 2000). The Lens model, discussed earlier, also offers a structure that can be used by practitioners to reflect upon clinical judgement/decision-making, identify information cues used to make inferences about patients, question how they know what they know, question their use of information cues in deciding interventions, and review the effectiveness of their judgement/decision-making in addressing the identified problem.
- **Patient and peer-aided judgement:** patient preference and expertise regarding their life choices (Binnie and Titchen 1999) that influence decisions through partnership with practitioners. It also refers to 'collaborative care' where practitioners from different disciplines work together in achieving common goals (ICN 2005a: 1). This provides an opportunity for observations to be compared, contrasted and collated within the team to enhance understanding of patients, clinical conditions, interventions used to manage them, and the local healthcare system. Patient and peer-aided judgement may be further enhanced through support from mentoring or clinical supervision.
- **System-aided judgement:** validated assessment tools, policies, procedures, clinical guidelines, conceptual/problem-solving frameworks, and decision analysis tools that contribute to an environment supporting nurses in clinical judgement and decision-making. The nursing process represents a long-standing example of a systematic framework through which judgements and decisions are made (Yura and Walsh 1973; ICN 2005b). Similarly, the 'Activities of living model' has been used extensively as a guide to assess a wide range of healthcare needs (Roper et al. 1990). Clinical guidelines developed by the then National Institute for

Clinical Excellence (NICE) gave access to research evidence from national projects to guide/update local procedures (Rycroft-Malone 2002). There is also a growing interest in applying decision analysis tools in nursing: Corcoran-Perry and Narayan (1995) described decision analysis applied to help a patient make an informed choice about hormone replacement therapy, identifying complications (osteoporosis, endometrial cancer) and survival risks for alternative options, and the patient's preferences regarding each outcome; O'Neill et al. (2004) developed computer software incorporating research evidence and expert opinion to guide nursing decisions; and Harbison (2006) advocates the application of Bayes' theorem to enhance understanding and use of statistics, as demonstrated in the earlier discussion.

- **Critical review of experiential and research evidence:** nurses 'stepping back' from practice and using critical thinking skills to evaluate their application of intuitive, reflective, patient and peer-aided, and system-aided judgement, plus seeking out and evaluating research studies that extend their understanding of nursing practice, clinical judgement, and research methods. Figure 5.3 shows this mode is positioned in the middle of the continuum and is a vital link between the world of clinical practice and the world of research. It is an important addition to the cognitive continuum because, without it, there is no mechanism to identify, critique, or apply research conducted elsewhere that is relevant to one's own practice. The skills needed include: question effectiveness of one's practice, question procedures, identify knowledge deficits, pose questions to address deficits, search, access, review, and apply findings to inform practice (Fleming and Fenton 2002). Ensuring 'evidence is made available and equipping staff with the skills to know how to evaluate and apply it' is essential for evidence-based clinical decisions (National Health Service Executive 1999: 8). Managerial support is, therefore, vital for staff development in critical thinking and research evaluation skills, plus work-based forums to discuss relevant studies and increase research utilization in practice areas (Maguire 1990; Mulhall and le May 2004). This mode also complements the role of advanced practitioners as knowledgeable critical thinkers (Chapter 2).
- **Action research and clinical audit:** identifying key principles and values underpinning an area of clinical practice and developing quality indicators to assess standards of practice. The practice area is then audited and strengths and weaknesses are identified. An action plan is drawn up to address weaknesses by identifying changes to be made, specifying criteria that indicate if change has occurred, agreeing who is responsible for the changes, agreeing a timeframe and then a repeat audit to evaluate implementation of the action plan. Review of audit procedures, principles and values then occurs, audit tools are revised as necessary, and the audit cycle repeated. This mode is an important addition to cognitive continuum theory in healthcare because, if there are organizational problems it will detract from care delivery, so action research and clinical audit are crucial to 'enhance the expertise of the system' (Paley 2004: 6). It also balances individual and organizational accountability in

the provision of healthcare and encourages all key stakeholders to participate and collaborate in implementing change (NICE 2002). It, therefore,
enhances effective integrated whole systems working in healthcare
(Chapter 3).

- **Qualitative research:** a commitment to eliciting, describing and interpreting experience from research participants'/respondents' perspectives
using of a range of methods to achieve this, including in-depth or semi-
structured interviews and observations in natural settings. This mode is
an important addition to the cognitive continuum applied to nursing
because the tasks (Figure 5.3) prompting judgement and decision-making
are patient-centred so it is vital to explore how patients feel about their
situation and care received. Attree (2001: 2–7) reported that patients
associated good care with being well informed 'they let you know what's
going on all the time and what they're going to do' whereas poor care
was perceived as routine, unrelated to needs, and impersonal. Grounded
theory was used to describe teenage women's experiences of maternity
services and understanding of motherhood (Price and Mitchell 2004).
Phenomenology was used to understand the lived experience of women
with HIV/AIDS (Beauregard and Solomon 2005). Hammond (1996) also
sought to 'encourage others to pursue the matter of the narrative as a
judgement process' (p. 200), suggesting that he is agreeable to qualitative
inquiry within the cognitive continuum.
- **Survey research:** systematically designing questionnaires or structured
interview schedules to seek answers to specific predetermined questions
via non-probability (convenience) or probability (random) sampling
of a target population. It aims to identify trends in attitudes, beliefs
or behaviour that are helpful in planning developments in healthcare
provision. Surveys may be targeted locally, nationally, or internationally,
for example: patient satisfaction feedback (Hays et al. 1998); nurses' use
of research information (Cullum 2002); oral hygiene practice by intensive
care unit staff (Furr *et al.* 2004); and current and projected future morbidity and mortality rates from infectious/parasitic diseases (WHO 2007).
Hence, 'The survey is a useful tool for policymakers' to plan for the future
(Hammond 1996: 3). It is, therefore, a valuable addition to the cognitive
continuum because surveys inform the strategic decisions that affect the
organization, management and delivery of healthcare provision.
- **Experimental research:** deducing hypotheses from theoretical assumptions and testing them in controlled environments by manipulating independent variables, measuring effects on dependent variables, analysing the
results, revising hypotheses where necessary, repeating the process until
cause and effect relationships are supported or refuted, and disseminating
findings. Experimental research includes: quasi-experiment, for example,
testing the effectiveness of a new hand hygiene procedure (Creedon 2005);
controlled trial, for example, testing the effects of a new drug against
a placebo by randomly allocating subjects to experimental and control
groups; and, scientific experiment, for example, developing the chemical
compound of a drug before it is trialled. Hammond's (1978) and Hamm's

(1988) modes 1–3 are, therefore, condensed into one 'experimental research' mode of practice in Standing's revised cognitive continuum.

Source of knowledge continuum

This shows an association between tacit knowledge and intuition, and between explicit knowledge and analysis (Eraut 2000). Intuitive judgement applies a very high level of tacit knowledge, experimental research applies a very high level of explicit knowledge, and the other seven modes combine the two: reflective, patient and peer-aided, and system-aided judgement have a higher proportion of tacit knowledge; critical review of experiential and research evidence has equal proportions of tacit and explicit knowledge; and, action research and clinical audit, qualitative and survey research have a higher proportion of explicit knowledge (Figure 5.3).

Interpret and apply ethical and professional codes of conduct continuum

Clinical judgement and decision-making are not simply a product of a system of tasks and a system of thinking interacting, they are also subject to a professional code of conduct specifying values that must be adhered to and applied, thereby influencing judgements and decisions (NMC 2008). The revised cognitive continuum shows nurses' 'live' professional accountability for their actions in face-to-face clinical practice. Where research methods are used as a mode of practice, ethical approval must be obtained prior to undertaking a study and if it is approved, then patients must be protected, including their right not to participate if they so choose. An ethical/professional continuum is, therefore, a necessary addition within the revised cognitive continuum as patients' human rights in nursing practice and/or research must be respected (ICN 1996). Furthermore, nurses often face challenging moral and ethical dilemmas regarding a patient's care (Esterhuizen and Kooyman 2001), and ethical and professional codes can be a resource to guide such decisions.

Correspondence and coherence competence in the nine modes of practice

These are included in the diagram of the revised cognitive continuum (Figure 5.3) to encourage self-assessment by practitioners in all nine modes of practice regarding two key questions: What have you observed about the patient that made you choose this mode of practice, and what observations can you make to check its effectiveness? (correspondence); and, What is the theoretical justification for choosing and applying this mode of practice rather than others? (coherence). Correspondence and coherence competence complement a professional code of conduct requiring nurses to act in the best interests of patients and justify their decisions (NMC 2008).

Reflective activity 5.3

This activity is intended to help you understand and apply cognitive continuum theory to your own practice. You will need pen and paper, Figure 5.3 (Revised cognitive continuum – nine practice modes), and be willing to use it to explore your clinical judgement and decision-making experience.

1. Identify a critical incident from your experience of clinical judgement and decision-making which you want to reflect on and explore. Refer to the left of Figure 5.3 and look at the range and examples of decision tasks. Identify the task/s associated with your critical incident.
2. Refer to the source of knowledge continuum at the bottom of Figure 5.3, identify whether you used tacit, explicit knowledge or a combination of the two in dealing with the situation and give examples of knowledge. Look, just above, at the cognitive range from intuition to analysis and decide whether you used analysis, intuition, or a mixture (if so, what proportions did you use?).
3. Look at the diagonal series of practice modes and explain which one/ones were used in dealing with the critical incident and why. Explain why you chose not to use alternative modes.
4. Refer to the right of Figure 5.3 and describe how much time you had to make a decision, the degree to which your judgement/decision-making process was open to scrutiny/checking by others, and whether or not you consciously controlled or manipulated the situation.
5. Look at the top of Figure 5.3 and reflect upon on ethical/moral issues or dilemmas associated with the critical incident, plus implications for practice in applying your professional code.
6. Self-assessment of your clinical judgement/decision-making skills: What did you observe about the patient that made you choose the mode/s of practice? What observations did you make to check their effectiveness? (Correspondence competence). What is the theoretical justification for choosing and applying the mode/s of practice rather than others? (Coherence competence).
7. In Figure 5.3 low structured tasks are linked to: tacit knowledge, intuition, intuitive judgement, little time for decision/lack of transparency/lack of conscious manipulation, individual 'on the spot' accountability, and more correspondence than coherence competence. High structured tasks are linked to: explicit knowledge, analysis, research experiments, enough time/visibility of decision-making process/conscious manipulation, shared professional/ethical responsibility, and more coherence than correspondence competence. Having reflected on a critical incident with the cognitive continuum, do you support or refute the above pattern of inter-related factors?
8. Are there any modes of practice that you need to develop further? How might you develop your intuitive and analytic judgement/decision-making skills? What can you do to monitor and enhance the relevance and rigour of your clinical judgement/decision-making? How useful is the cognitive continuum as a tool to guide, examine, explain and develop decision-making skills?

Potential applications of the revised cognitive continuum – nine modes of practice

1. **Practice guide** – framework that integrates the theory and practice of clinical judgement and decision-making in nursing and interprofessional healthcare to enhance knowledge and skills needed to benefit patients and justify decisions. Promote understanding of the choices available in matching patient-centred decision tasks to the most appropriate practice mode. Raise awareness of errors of judgement and how to minimize them. Validate observational skills and reflective practice in healthcare as a viable form of evidence regarding clinical contexts. Encourage research appreciation and evaluation in evidence-based practice. Apply ethical values from NMC or other relevant professional code of Conduct to judgements and decisions. Develop correspondence competence to ensure all interventions benefit patients, and coherence competence to ensure that the logic and rational for decisions can be explained and defended.

2. **Educational tool** – in-depth understanding of contrasting decision theories, the development of cognitive continuum theory, and its application in medicine, nursing or allied health professions. Workshops for participants to relate the nine modes of practice to their clinical experience and raise awareness of the range of decision tasks encountered, the strategies used to manage them, and evaluation of the different sources of knowledge that inform them. Self-assessment framework to identify strengths and weaknesses in maintaining a personal/professional portfolio and identifying development needs. Device to assist mentoring and clinical supervision in reviewing experiences of clinical judgement and decision-making, identifying any knowledge or skills deficits, and addressing them.

3. **Managerial tool** – mechanism to support a work-based learning culture that facilitates reflective practice and the application of research evidence to patient-centred care. Promote the use of clinical audit to enhance the effectiveness of the system of healthcare. Create a work-based forum to discuss relevant research studies that help to question and inform local practice. Review and develop resources to support system-aided judgement including policies, procedures, guidelines, assessment strategies and decision analysis tools. Incorporate correspondence and coherence competence in criteria for staff appraisal. Identify/address staff development needs in clinical judgement and decision-making.

4. **Research guide** – interpretation of cognitive continuum theory that is inclusive of a wide range of research methods. Promote the development and application of critical appraisal skills in literature searching, identifying relevant studies, evaluating them and applying what has been learnt to enhance understanding of a practice area. Encourage new research projects in exploring clinical judgement and decision-making in nursing and interprofessional healthcare.

Summary

Cognitive continuum theory combines contrasting intuitive/experiential and analytic/rational decision theories and matches a wide range of decision tasks to a variety of judgement/decision-making skills best suited to address them. Understanding the strengths and weaknesses of both intuitive/experiential and analytic/rational judgement/decision-making enables them to be applied more effectively. The revised cognitive continuum promotes awareness of a variety of patient-centred judgement decision tasks and identifies nine modes of practice to address them. This has five new modes of practice (reflective judgement, critical review of experiential and research evidence, action research and clinical audit, qualitative research, and survey research) providing a broader range of evidence-based options than before. Practitioners' skill in applying each mode of practice is evaluated regarding their demonstration of correspondence competence (practical outcome of care) and coherence competence (logical process of decision-making). Detailed examples of applying theory to practice were presented, supplemented by reflective activities that encouraged readers to reflect on practice and enhance their judgement/decision-making skills.

Cognitive continuum theory supports the synthesis of reflective and evidence-based practice portrayed by the Matrix model (Chapter 1) and the development of advanced practitioners as knowledgeable, critical thinkers (Chapter 2). The interaction between a patient-centred system of decision tasks and a system of cognitive tactics that includes auditing healthcare systems, complements whole systems theory (Chapter 3). The source of knowledge continuum supports the need to develop both tacit and explicit knowledge via informal and formal learning (Chapter 4). Collectively, this provides a broad theoretical framework with which to interpret the following accounts of advanced practitioners' clinical judgement and decision-making in healthcare contexts.

Key points

- Cognitive continuum theory relates low/high structured decision tasks to a range of intuitive and analytic modes in order to continually match decision tactics to changing practice priorities.
- In the Lens model, intuition involves: perceive many observable information cues; 'weigh up' which underlying problem they allude to; and apply this to inform judgement/decision-making.
- Ecological validity assesses relevance of cues/signs in truly representing underlying condition.
- In Bayes' theorem, analysis involves: determine national base rates; test local sample, analyse true/false positive/negative results; and predict statistical probability to inform decision-making.
- Scientific validity assesses rigour in testing cause/effect relations when manipulating variables.

- Low structured decision tasks e.g. check how a patient feels, prompt greater intuition, apply tacit knowledge, use pattern recognition of information cues, are not auditable, and are quick.
- Highly structured decision tasks e.g. develop new medicine, prompt greater analysis, apply explicit knowledge, establish cause/effect relationships, are auditable, and take a lot more time.
- Nine modes of practice = intuitive, reflective, patient/peer-aided, system-aided *judgement*; critical review experiential/research evidence; action/audit, qualitative, survey, experimental *research*.
- All nine modes of practice can be evaluated regarding practitioners' correspondence competence (practical benefits to patients) and coherence competence (logical/theoretical justification).

References

Attree, M. (2001) Patients' and relatives' experience of 'good' and 'not so good' quality care. *Journal of Advanced Nursing,* 33(4): 456–66.

Beauregard, C. and Solomon, P. (2005) Understanding the experience of HIV/AIDS for women: implications for occupational therapy. *Journal for Occupational Therapy,* 72(2): 113–20.

Bell, D.E., Raiffa, H. and Tversky, A. (1995) Descriptive, normative and prescriptive interactions in decision making, in D.E. Bell, H. Raiffa, H. and A. Tversky (eds) *Decision Making.* Cambridge: Cambridge University Press, pp. 9–30.

Benner, P. (1984) *From Novice to Expert.* Menlo Park, CA: Addison-Wesley.

Benner, P., Tanner, C.A. and Chesla, C.A. (1996) *Expertise in Nursing Practice.* New York: Springer.

Benner, P. and Wrubel, J. (1989) *The Primacy of Caring: Stress and coping in health and illness.* Menlo Park, CA: Addison-Wesley.

Binnie, A. and Titchen, A. (1999) *Freedom to Practise: The development of patient-centred nursing.* Oxford: Butterworth-Heinemann.

Brehmer, B. and Joyce, C.R.B. (eds) (1988) *Human Judgment: The SJT view.* Elsevier: Amsterdam.

Brunswik, E. (1943) Organismic achievement and environmental probability. *Psychological Review,* 50: 255–72.

Brunswik, E. (1956) *Perception and the Representative Design of Psychological Experiments,* 2nd edn. Berkeley: University of California Press.

Cancer Research UK (2009) Breast cancer – UK incidence statistics. http://info.cancerresearchuk.org/cancerstats/types/breast/incidence

Cooksey, R. (1996) *Judgment Analysis: Theory, methods, and applications.* San Diego: Academic Press.

Corcoran-Perry, S. and Narayan, S. (1995) Clinical decision making, in M. Snyder and M.P. Mirr (eds) *Advanced Nursing Practice.* New York: Springer, pp. 69–91.

Creedon, S.A. (2005) Health workers' hand decontamination practices: compliance with recommended guidelines. *Journal of Advanced Nursing,* 51(3): 208–16.

Cullum, N. (2002) *Nurses' Use of Research Information in Clinical Decision Making: A descriptive and analytical study.* London: Department of Health. http://www.dh.gov.uk/Policyandguidance/Researchanddevelopment/AZ/ Promotingimplementationresearchfindings/DH4001837: 2/07/2006.

Dawes, R.M., Faust, D. and Meehl, P.E. (1989) Clinical versus actuarial judgment. *Science*, 243: 1668–73.

Dowie, J. (1993) Clinical decision analysis: background and introduction, in H. Llewelyn and A. Hopkins (eds) *Analysing How We Reach Clinical Decisions*. London: Royal College of Physicians, pp. 7–26.

Edwards, W. (1954) The theory of decision making. *Psychological Bulletin*, 41: 380–417.

Edwards, W., Lindman, H., and Savage, J. (1963) Bayesian statistical inference for psychological research. *Psychological Review*, 70: 193–242.

Eraut, M. (2000) Non-formal learning and tacit knowledge in professional work. *British Journal of Educational Psychology*, 70: 113–36.

Esterhuizen, P. and Kooyman, A. (2001) Empowering moral decision making in nurses. *Nurse Education Today*, 21: 640–7.

Fleming, K. and Fenton, M. (2002) Making sense of research evidence to inform decision making, in C. Thompson and D. Dowding (eds) *Clinical Decision Making and Judgement in Nursing*. Edinburgh: Churchill Livingstone, pp. 109–29.

Furr, L., Allen Binkley, C.J., McCurren, C. and Carrico, R. (2004) Factors affecting the quality of oral care in intensive care units. *Journal of Advanced Nursing*, 48(5): 454–62.

Gigerenzer, G. (1991) How to make cognitive illusions disappear: beyond 'heuristics and biases'. *European Review of Social Psychology*, 2: 83–115.

Hamm, R.M. (1988) Clinical intuition and clinical analysis: expertise and the cognitive continuum, in J. Dowie and A. Elstein (eds) *Professional Judgement: A reader in clinical decision making*. Cambridge: Cambridge University Press, pp. 78–109.

Hammond, K.R. (1955) Probabilistic functioning and the clinical method. *Psychological Review*, 62: 255–62.

Hammond, K.R. (1978) Toward increasing competence of thought in public policy formation, in K.R. Hammond (ed.) *Judgment and Decision in Public Policy Formation*. Boulder, CO: Westview Press, pp. 11–32.

Hammond, K.R. (1996) *Human Judgment and Social Policy: Irreducible uncertainty, inevitable error, unavoidable injustice*. New York: Oxford University Press.

Hammond, K.R. (2007) *Beyond Rationality: The search for wisdom in a troubled time*. New York: Oxford University Press.

Harbison, J. (2006) Clinical judgement in the interpretation of evidence: a Bayesian approach. *Journal of Clinical Nursing*, 15: 1489–97.

Hays, R.D., Brown, J.A., Spritzer, K.L., Dixon, W.J. and Brook, R.H. (1998) Satisfaction with health care provided by 48 physician group. *Archives of Internal Medicine*, 158: 785–790.

Heider, F. (1944) Social perception and phenomenal causality. *Psychological Review*, 51: 358–74.

Heider, F. (1958) *The Psychology of Interpersonal Relations*. New York: John Wiley and Sons.

International Council of Nurses (ICN) (1996) *Ethical Guidelines for Nursing Research*. Geneva: ICN.

International Council of Nurses (ICN) (2005a) *The ICN Definition of Nursing*. Geneva: ICN. http://www.icn.ch/definition.htm (accessed 12 January 2007).

International Council of Nurses (ICN) (2005b) *International Classification of Nursing Practice [ICNP] Version 1.0 Book Chapter 4 – The 7-Axis Model*. Geneva: ICN. http://www.icn.ch/icnp_v1book_ch4.htm (accessed 5 January 2007).

Johns, C. (2000) *Becoming a Reflective Practitioner.* Oxford: Blackwell Science.

Kahneman, D., Slovic, P. and Tversky, A. (eds) (1982) *Judgment under Uncertainty: Heuristics and biases.* Cambridge: Cambridge University Press.

Kahneman, D. and Tversky, A. (1979) Prospect theory: An analysis of decision under risk. *Econometrica,* XLVII, 263–91.

Knill-Jones, R. (1993) The role of Bayes' theorem in diagnosis, prediction and decision making, in H. Llewelyn and A. Hopkins (eds) *Analysing How We Reach Clinical Decisions.* London: Royal College of Physicians.

Lamond, D. and Thompson, C. (2000) Intuition and analysis in decision making and choice. *Journal of Nursing Scholarship,* 32(4): 411–14.

Lauri, S., Salantera, S., Chalmers, K. et al. (2001) An exploratory study of clinical decision-making in five countries. *Journal of Nursing Scholarship,* 33: 83–90.

Maguire, J.M. (1990) Putting nursing research findings into practice: research utilization as an aspect of the management of change, *Journal of Advanced Nursing,* 15: 614–20.

Mayers, C.P. (1977) *Pathology,* 2nd edn. London: Hodder and Stoughton.

Muir Gray, J.A. (1999) *Evidence-based Healthcare: How to make health policy and management decisions.* Edinburgh: Churchill Livingstone.

Mulhall, A. and le May, A. (2004) Reviewing the case for critical appraisal skills training. *Clinical Effectiveness in Nursing,* 8: 101–10.

National Health Service Executive (NHSE) (1999) *Clinical Governance: Quality in the new NHS.* Leeds: NHSE.

National Institute for Clinical Excellence (2002) *Principles for Best Practice in Clinical Audit.* Oxford: Radcliffe Medical Press.

Nursing and Midwifery Council (NMC) (2008) *The NMC Code of Professional Conduct: Standards for conduct, performance and ethics.* London: NMC.

O'Neill, E.S., Dluhy, N.M., Fortier, P.J. and Michel, H.E. (2004) Knowledge acquisition, synthesis, and validation: A model for decision support systems. *Journal of Advanced Nursing,* 47(2): 134–42.

Paley, J. (2004) Clinical cognition and embodiment. *International Journal of Nursing Studies,* 41(1): 1–13.

Price, S. and Mitchell, M. (2004) Teenagers' experiences of maternity services. *Evidence Based Midwifery,* 2(2): 66–70.

Roper, N., Logan, W.W. and Tierney, A.J. (1990) *The Elements of Nursing,* 3rd edn. Edinburgh: Churchill Livingstone.

Rycroft-Malone, J. (2002) Clinical guidelines, in C. Thompson and D. Dowding (eds) *Clinical Decision Making and Judgement in Nursing.* Edinburgh: Churchill Livingstone.

Savage, L.J. (1954) *The Foundations of Statistics.* New York: Wiley.

Schön, D.A. (1987) *Educating the Reflective Practitioner: Towards a new design for teaching and learning in the professions.* San Francisco: Jossey-Bass.

Simon, H.E. (1957) *Models of Man: Social and rational.* New York: Wiley.

Standing, M. (2005) Perceptions of clinical decision-making skills on a developmental journey from student to staff nurse. PhD thesis, University of Kent, Canterbury.

Standing, M. (2007) Clinical decision-making skills on the developmental journey from student to Registered Nurse: a longitudinal inquiry, *Journal of Advanced Nursing,* 60(3): 257–69.

Standing, M. (2008) Clinical judgement and decision-making in nursing – nine modes of practice in a revised cognitive continuum. *Journal of Advanced Nursing,* 62(1): 124–34.

Taylor, B. (2000) *Reflective Practice: A guide for nurses and midwives.* Buckingham: Open University Press.

Thompson, C., Cullum, N., McCaughan, D., Sheldon, T., and Raynor, P. (2004) Nurses, information use, and clinical making – the real world potential for evidence-based decisions in nursing, *Evidence-based Nursing*, 7: 68–72.

World Health Organization (2007) *Ten Statistical Highlights in Global Public Health.* http://www.who.int/whosis/highlight10.png (accessed 17 March 2007).

Yudkowsky, E.S. (2003) *An Intuitive Explanation of Bayesian Reasoning.* http://yudkowsky.net/bayes.html (accessed 1 November 2007).

Yura, H. and Walsh, M.B. (1973) *The Nursing Process: Assessing, planning, implementing, evaluating.*, 2nd edn. New York: Appleton-Century-Crofts.

6 Prioritizing decisions during the patient journey

Roger Goldsmith and Michael Standing

Overview

In this chapter the concept of a 'patient journey' is used to highlight each stage of care delivery and associated clinical decision-making priorities in a case study of an actual patient's care. The setting for the case study is a nurse-led minor injury unit (MIU) and the discussion focuses on the role of an emergency nurse practitioner (ENP) in diagnosing and treating a patient's broken hand bone. An overview is given of health policy influencing the organization and delivery of emergency care. Prioritization is discussed in relation to: provision of a 24-hour emergency service, compliance with government-prescribed health targets, a triage system of assessing and attending to patients with more urgent needs first, and in deciding what intervention to use and why. Each of the theoretical perspectives discussed in Chapters 1–5 is applied to clinical judgement/decision-making within the case study. The focus on emergency care enables a complete cycle of decision-making from admission to discharge to be discussed and highlights the autonomy and responsibility of an ENP. Reflective activities are incorporated throughout the chapter to encourage readers to relate the content to clinical decision-making priorities and the 'patient journey' in their own area of practice.

Objectives

- Describe the concept of a 'patient journey' and identify care priorities in each of its stages
- Categorize case study decisions by applying the 10 perceptions of clinical decision-making
- Appreciate how collaborative networking contributes to effective whole systems in a MIU
- Relate identified advanced practitioner attributes to a range of decisions in the case study
- Describe proactive, critical and reflective work-based lifelong learning in decision-making
- Apply cognitive continuum theory to stages/priorities of the patient journey in the case study
- Engage in reflective activities relating chapter content to care priorities in own practice area

Prioritizing the provision of emergency care

Maintaining the provision of accessible emergency care, free at the point of delivery, remains a political and social priority in the ongoing review and reform of the National Health Service (NHS) (Tippins and Evans 2007). The Department of Health's ten-year strategy 'Reforming Emergency Care' (DH 2001) initiated organizational and managerial change to improve the efficiency and effectiveness of the service, optimize use of sustainable resources, identify minimum standards, and set targets to achieve high quality care delivery. One target stated that, by the end of 2004, no patient should spend more than four hours in an accident and emergency department (A&E) or other emergency setting from time of admission to time of transfer or discharge home (DH 2001). Government policy and health targets therefore impact on ENPs' clinical judgement and decision-making in the management and delivery of emergency care.

The management of minor injuries forms part of emergency care provision in the United Kingdom. Minor injury units (MIUs) may be attached to A&E departments or function independently of major trauma services. MIUs are usually nurse-led and focus mainly on assessing and treating patients with a wide variety of non-life-threatening injuries such as cuts, abrasions, bruises, sprains, closed fractures, superficial burns, or foreign body in the eye and some treat acute symptoms of minor illnesses (Alberti 2007). The treatment of minor injuries depends upon the knowledge and clinical expertise of MIU personnel, adequate equipment and support services, and effective management of resources. Patients accessing the service can be of any age and from any part of society, rich or poor, and private health insurance is not needed to receive care (Goldsmith and Lumsden 2008).

Prioritizing decisions during the 'patient journey'

Analysing and evaluating the clinical judgement and decision-making of advanced practitioners are important to enhance patients' experience of care, facilitate ongoing professional development, and review compliance with government health targets. The notion of NHS users undertaking a journey has stimulated monitoring of the 'patient journey' to facilitate meeting health targets (DH 2005a); improve access, increase efficiency, reduce waste in public health services (DH 2005b); and enable audit of the patient experience (DH 2005c). The concept of a patient journey is used to structure care delivery and decision priorities from booking in to discharge in a MIU (Table 6.1).

The stages of the patient journey in Table 6.1 reflect government health targets regarding access to 24-hour emergency care and the need to complete it within 4 hours. The priorities associated with each stage highlight ENPs' leadership responsibility for coordinating care delivery in a nurse led MIU. The ENP's own clinical expertise is focussed mainly between stages 4–10 in

Table 6.1 Stages of the 'patient journey' and priorities in a minor injury unit (MIU)

Stage	Description	Priorities
1	**Booking in**	Maintain 24-hour MIU service available for public to self-refer
2	**Triage assessment**	Assess injury and decide if it is a low, medium or high priority Decide if injury is treatable or if urgent transfer to A&E is needed
3	**Initial treatment**	Give first aid to prevent further harm and reduce suffering
4	**ENP consultation**	Elicit the patient's history of injury and description of symptoms
5	**Examination**	Systematically observe and assess extent and effects of injury
6	**Investigation**	Authorize tests to confirm/eliminate pathophysiology, as needed
7	**Review investigation**	Carefully analyse test results and consider their implications
8	**Diagnosis**	Collate assessment/test results to facilitate accurate diagnosis
9	**Treatment**	Plan/implement action to promote healing and relieve suffering
10	**Health promotion**	Advise on wound/injury management and preventative health
11	**Documentation**	Record care/Letter to GP/Follow-up referral/Patient evaluation
12	**Discharge**	Whole process completed and patient discharged within 4 hours

accurately assessing/diagnosing, effectively treating patients' injuries, and giving health promotion advice. Enabling patients to successfully negotiate the patient journey from booking in to discharge is dependent on ENPs' application of effective clinical judgement/decision-making skills.

Reflective activity 6.1

This activity is intended to help you relate the concept of a patient journey to clinical decision-making priorities in your own area of nursing/interprofessional healthcare practice.

1. Refer to Table 6.1 and copy the headings on a sheet of paper to compile your own table.
2. How would you describe the patient journey in your area of practice? How many stages can you identify? What are they called? What are the priorities

associated with each stage? Please write your responses in the appropriate columns of your table.

3. To what extent do your identified stages of the patient journey reflect current health policy?
4. What decisions are you responsible for? Which stages of the patient journey do they relate to?
5. What methods do you use to prioritize care between one patient and another?
6. How do you prioritize what care to give to each individual patient?

Professional profile

I (Roger) have 25 years experience in emergency care, am a university lecturer in nursing, and a part-time Emergency Nurse Practitioner (ENP). The case study relates to my ENP practice in a nurse-led minor injury unit (MIU) providing 24-hour care at a busy general hospital whose accident and emergency department was closed in a reorganization of major trauma services. The case study was explored during my reflections on practice as part of my obligation to create and maintain a personal professional portfolio and demonstrate and apply relevant lifelong learning.

Case study in a minor injury unit

'Miss Cartwright' (pseudonym), a 36-year-old physiotherapist, attended the MIU after falling while out jogging. She was muddy, dishevelled, anxious, tearful, and complained of severe pain in her right hand. Miss Cartwright was booked in by the receptionist and then assessed as a high priority by the triage nurse who also gave painkilling tablets and placed her arm in a sling. She was then seen by the ENP who examined her hand and requested an X-ray showing a comminuted (multiple) fracture of right hand fourth metacarpal bone (ring finger).

The ENP telephoned the duty orthopaedic surgeon, based at another hospital, to check whether surgery was indicated but it was not considered necessary. A plaster cast was applied to the right hand and forearm and Miss Cartwright was discharged home with a fracture clinic appointment.

Perceptions of clinical decision-making and patient journey stages/priorities

Each of the ten clinical decision-making themes discussed in Chapter 1 can be applied to the 'patient journey' stages and priorities (Table 6.1) in the case study. The 'prioritizing' theme is the main focus because of the urgent nature of emergency care. This is reflected in the structure of the service, freely available on a 24-hour basis to any member of the public who judges or is judged that they need urgent healthcare. Self-referral to emergency care (Stage 1) without needing medical referral saves time, and is essential to reduce morbidity/mortality rates and alleviate suffering through early assessment and intervention. While the MIU does not cater for life-threatening injuries, the same principles apply: applying a triage system to prioritize care according to greatest clinical need (Tippins and Evans 2007); and fast access to assessment, investigations, review of investigations, diagnosis and treatment (Stages 2–9), for example, to relieve Miss Cartwright's distress and pain as quickly as possible, promote healing of the fourth metacarpal in her right hand, reduce the risk of complications arising, and contribute to her full and speedy recovery.

The 'collaborative' theme is evident in gaining all patients' cooperation and understanding of the triage system where being first in the queue did not guarantee being seen first. Each member of the MIU team made an important contribution to Miss Cartwright's collective care. I was assisted by the radiography department in providing clear evidence of a fracture, and by the orthopaedic surgeon in offering expert opinion to guide my choice of treatment. Miss Cartwright also actively contributed to her care by giving a detailed account of her injury, agreeing to a clinical examination despite her discomfort, responding to advice on how to manage her injury (Stage 10), and attending follow-up fracture clinic appointments. Collaboration between MIU, general practitioner and orthopaedic team also facilitated continuity of care beyond emergency treatment to promote Miss Cartwright's full recovery and the resumption of her work and leisure activities (Stages 11–12).

The 'experience and intuition' theme is applicable although more difficult to quantify. After working in emergency care for many years I had acquired experiential knowledge and practical skills in assessing and treating upper limb injuries. This was helpful in Miss Cartwright's case as I had a cumulative 'memory bank' of patients presenting with similar problems which made it easier for me to recognize the significance of her signs or symptoms and understand how to intervene. Similarly, the 'confidence' theme was linked with experience as I was accustomed to dealing with pressure working in busy accident and emergency and minor injury units. This enabled me to remain calm and focused when assessing each patient which was important in putting Miss Cartwright at ease and gaining her trust in me. My confidence in decision-making was also linked to the 'systematic' theme which enabled me to discover a sound evidence base to support diagnosis and treatment. This included applying a structured problem solving approach within the consultation process to elicit relevant history, the physical examination of the right hand to identify impaired function, and the review of X-ray investigations to carefully inspect each bone and joint for anatomical defects. The 'observation' theme dovetailed with applying a systematic approach as I had to be attentive and observant in judging Miss Cartwright's level of pain, appearance and feel of her right hand, appearance of the different X-ray views, and in checking that the plaster cast fitted properly.

The 'standardized' theme was applied in the policies, procedures and clinical guidelines used in the MIU. This influences how minor injuries are defined and the inclusion and exclusion criteria concerning admission to the MIU or transfer to an A&E unit dealing with major trauma. Life-threatening or serious injuries and acute illnesses associated with severe shock, haemorrhage, loss of consciousness, chest pain, breathing difficulty and compound fractures need to be transferred directly to A&E. Locally agreed standardized guidelines identifying criteria to adhere to when carrying out procedures also influenced Miss Cartwright's care in the MIU including: the triage system of prioritizing care; an assessment tool for upper limb injuries that complemented my systematic examination of her right hand (Bickley 2007); and administration of painkillers by nurses in the absence of medical personnel. Furthermore, the computerized timing, tracking and record keeping comply with national standards or health targets requiring emergency care to be completed and patient discharged within four hours (Stage 12).

The 'reflective' theme is evident throughout Miss Cartwright's care in consciously weighing up, cross-referencing varied information sources, reaching conclusions based on available evidence and making diagnostic and treatment decisions ('reflection-in-action'). Documenting the care given also provided a brief opportunity to look back and think about what had transpired ('reflection-on-action') before attending to the next patient (Schön 1987). In a sense there was a reflective aspect in each of the other themes, for example, I had to think about how I applied a systematic problem solving approach or standardized procedures to Miss Cartwright's individual care needs. Continual reflection-in-action also serves as a safeguard to question assumptions and respond to new information or changing circumstances, for example, when I discovered Miss Cartwright had sustained a comminuted fracture I was aware this could be more difficult to mend than a simple fracture and so decided to double-check my proposed treatment with the orthopaedic surgeon. Writing this chapter also provides an opportunity for more in-depth reflection-on-action in looking back, describing, analysing and evaluating judgement and decisions in Miss Cartwright's care.

The 'ethical sensitivity' theme was applicable in recognizing the pain and distress Miss Cartwright was suffering due to her injury and taking care not to make it any worse ('non-maleficence'), for example, I asked her to tell me to stop if I caused her too much pain when examining her hand and a wheelchair was provided to prevent her falling when she complained of dizziness. The MIU team were committed to taking positive steps to improve her sense of well-being ('beneficence'), for example, the triage nurse recognized she needed pain relief and gave her analgesic tablets and I checked with the orthopaedic surgeon that applying a plaster cast was the best treatment. I was obliged to respect patients' basic human rights of self-determination ('autonomy'), for example, in gaining Miss Cartwright's informed consent to be examined and treated, and sharing information with her including showing her the X-rays and explaining the findings (Fletcher et al. 1995; Maude and Hawley 2007; Dimond 2008; NMC 2008). I was also aware of the need to demonstrate consistency and fairness in the way patients perceived others to be treated, for example, following triage assessment Miss Cartwright was seen before other patients because her injury was more serious and not because she happened to be a fellow health professional.

The 'accountability' theme was evident in carrying out both my clinical and managerial roles in the nurse-led MIU. I had to be able to justify or defend judgement and decisions directly to the patient, contractually to my NHS trust employers, and professionally to the Nursing and Midwifery Council (NMC 2008). I was accountable for conducting a comprehensive examination of Miss Cartwright, requesting and reviewing X-ray investigations, reaching an accurate evidence-based diagnosis, recognizing the limits of my own expertise to seek advice from an orthopaedic surgeon, planning and implementing effective treatment, and organizing appropriate after-care arrangements. The importance of developing and applying a high level of clinical skill in carrying out these activities is underlined by instances where patients' injuries have been missed, a head injury, for example, and they have been discharged from emergency care without the required treatment with serious, sometimes fatal, consequences. I knew Miss Cartwright had sustained a fall so I checked whether she had bumped her head by asking her directly about it, looking for visible signs, and asking if she could recall everything that happened as this would help to highlight any loss of consciousness. As the senior ENP in the nurse-led MIU I also had responsibility for effective operational management including supporting other team members; ensuring local policies were complied with, for example, preventing Miss Cartwright's boyfriend using his mobile phone to photograph X-rays; and ensuring all patients attending the unit were treated inside four hours according to the government target.

Perceptions of clinical decision-making associated with registered nurses (Standing 2007) can therefore be used to describe or review decision priorities associated with ENP advanced practice and the patient journey in a nurse-led MIU. The perceptions of clinical decision-making can also be cross-referenced against the personal characteristics associated with advanced practitioners.

Characteristics of advanced practitioners and patient journey stages/priorities

The personal characteristics of advanced practitioners (Chapter 2) correspond with the above perceptions of clinical decision-making and they can be combined in analysing the case study with reference to stages of the patient journey, as illustrated by Table 6.2.

Table 6.2 cross-references personal characteristics of advanced practitioners with perceptions of clinical decision-making skills indicating that they are central to advanced practice. This view is reinforced by examples from the case study linking these characteristics and skills to ENP practice and stages of

Table 6.2 Linking advanced practitioners' personal characteristics and perceptions of clinical decision-making to case study of ENP practice within nurse-led MIU

Advanced practitioner characteristics	Perceptions of clinical decision–making	Case study examples of ENP practice in nurse-led MIU related to stages of the patient journey (see Table 6.1)
Knowledgeable	Experience and intuition, systematic	Intuition from previous experience re. possible nature of hand injury confirmed by systematic assessment and investigation (Stages 4–8)
Understands system	Prioritizing, standardized	Triage system gave patient's care high priority re. greater clinical need. Met health targets re. access/care duration 4 hours (Stages 1–2 and 12)
Visionary	Observation, reflective	Attend to signs, symptoms, X-ray results, and recognize treatment implications. Reflect on professional development (Stages 9 and 11)
Risk taker	Prioritizing, accountability	Risk of exacerbating pain during examination outweighed by need to determine extent of injury and mitigated by painkillers (Stage 5)
Good interpersonal abilities	Collaborative, ethical sensitivity	Empathizing with patient re. anxiety about injury. Effective communication, teamwork with MIU/hospital/community personnel (Stage 4)
Confident and motivated	Confidence, experience and intuition	Enjoy challenge of helping patient in time of need, working in pressurized environment. Not afraid to seek orthopaedic advice (Stages 7–9)
Creative critical thinker	Reflective, collaborative	Helped design, review and develop clinical guidelines and procedures used in MIU through interprofessional collaboration (Stage 11)
Goodness	Ethical sensitivity, accountability	Commitment to caring: relieve patient's pain and distress, treat fracture effectively, maximize chance of a full recovery (Stages 3 and 9)
Autonomous	Accountability, systematic	ENP leadership of nurse-led MIU and expertise to assess, diagnose and prescribe treatment for injuries using advanced skills (Stages 1–12)

the patient journey. Prioritizing is directly related to characteristics of 'understands system' (in terms of triage, access, and 4-hour health target), and 'risk taker' (in terms of potentially causing patient discomfort during physical examination in order to assess the severity of injury). All advanced practitioner characteristics and perceptions of clinical decision-making are, collectively, related to priorities associated with the stages of the patient journey (Table 6.1) in the case study.

Reflective activity 6.2

This activity is intended to help you to relate characteristics of advanced practitioners to stages of the patient journey, perceptions of clinical decision-making, and prioritizing care in your practice.

1. Refer to Table 6.2 and draw up your own table using the same column headings and in the first column list the identified advanced practitioner characteristics (as in Table 6.2).
2. Identify and reflect on a patient case study in which you are/were involved in providing the care.
3. In the third column give examples of how you apply each advanced practitioner characteristic to your case study and identify which stages of the patient journey your examples relate to.
4. In the second column identify which perceptions of clinical decision-making you think are being applied (this is dependent on your examples so it might not be the same order as Table 6.2).
5. Where a 'prioritizing' perception is identified, reflect on why case study examples required this and how related advanced practitioner characteristics helped to inform clinical decision-making.

The application of the ENP's clinical expertise in prioritizing the diagnosis and treatment of injuries takes place in stages 4–9 of the patient journey (Table 6.1). It is dependent on establishing a structured therapeutic relationship with patients using 'good interpersonal abilities' which are also desirable characteristics of advanced practitioners (Table 6.2) in their consultations with patients.

A professional consultation model identifies five practitioner tasks (Neighbour 2005) and examples are provided of how I interpreted these tasks as an ENP in the case study, as follows:

1. **Connecting:** Has the practitioner developed an effective rapport with the patient? As a fellow health professional I empathized with Miss Cartwright's anxiety about how her injury would affect her job as a physiotherapist and I understood she was in pain.
2. **Summarizing:** Can the practitioner demonstrate to the patient sufficient understanding of the help needed? (Practitioner elicits and listens to patient responses; the patient's ideas, feelings, concerns and expectations

are explored and acknowledged; and practitioner assesses, diagnoses, explains, negotiates and agrees treatment with patient.) My main role at this point was as a detective combining open and closed questions to enable both general exploration and specific probing to elicit the cause and extent of the injury (Shah 2005a, 2005b; Redsell and Hastings 2006; Moss 2008). For example, I asked 'How did you come to injure your hand?' and, 'Did your hand hit the ground?' The physical examination was conducted as gently as possible and this indicated an X-ray of the right hand was needed. Miss Cartwright was shown the X-ray of her broken metacarpal and informed that it had been seen by an orthopaedic surgeon who recommended a plaster cast rather than surgical fixation.

3. **Handing over:** Has the patient accepted the agreed management plan? The broken metacarpal was in the patient's dominant hand and as a physiotherapist her hands are her livelihood, so she had reason to refuse the proposed treatment and request a surgical option at another hospital if she wished. She consented to having a plaster cast applied.

4. **Safety netting:** What if problems or complications occur? (The practitioner needs to be able to: predict what could happen if things go well; discuss how to manage an unexpected turn of events; and consider contingency plans.) I informed Miss Cartwright that union of the broken bone should occur in 10–12 weeks and she would be monitored at the out-patients fracture clinic in the meantime to minimize the danger of complications (infection, non-union, deformity, reduced finger grip) and ensure healing occurs. Miss Cartwright was advised to return to the unit at any time if the plaster cast got too tight or her fingers became swollen, blue, or numb as the plaster cast might need replacing to prevent complications arising from possible impaired circulation. 'How to care for upper limb injuries' and 'How to care for your plaster' information leaflets were given to reinforce verbal advice.

5. **Housekeeping:** Is the practitioner in a good condition to receive the next patient? (Are there any outstanding issues the practitioner needs to deal with before seeing another patient? Is the practitioner ready and able to concentrate on helping the next patient?) I checked Miss Cartwright's plaster cast fitted comfortably, ensured referral letters and an out-patients appointment had been made, and recorded the care that had been given via clear, concise factual notes to enable effective communication (Purcell 2003; Kettenbach 2009).

'Connecting', 'summarizing', and 'handing over' tasks in Neighbour's consultation model are linked to triage nurses' role in stages 2–3 of the patient journey (and related priorities) and to ENPs' role in stages 4–9. 'Safety netting' and 'housekeeping' tasks are linked to ENPs' role in stages 10–12. Each advanced practitioner characteristic (Table 6.2) is applied in the five tasks of Neighbour's consultation model which enable ENP clinical expertise to diagnose and treat injuries. Neighbour's model accommodates systematic problem solving within a structure that emphasizes interpersonal engagement and collaborative decision-making with the patient, and, anticipating consequences of planned actions. This facilitates recognition of different levels of prioritizing in terms of resolving immediate concerns, having a strategy ready to tackle possible future complications, and always respecting the autonomy of patients in and facilitating their contribution to clinical decision-making.

Reflective activity 6.3

This activity is intended to help you relate Neighbour's consultation model to your area of practice. Please identify/reflect on an example of your assessment or treatment of patient.

1. Connecting – How did you establish/maintain rapport with the patient during the consultation?
2. Summarizing – How did you demonstrate understanding of the problem and possible solution?
3. Handing over – How did you check that the patient was agreeable to the proposed care?
4. Safety netting – What could have gone wrong? What contingency plans did you have for this?
5. Housekeeping – What details did you need to attend to in order to prepare for the next patient?
6. Do you find that Neighbour's five tasks help to clarify patient-centred current and future priorities?
7. How might you apply Neighbour's consultation model to your clinical decision-making in future?

The contribution of team members supports ENPs' application of clinical expertise in consultations with patients, and in achieving successful outcomes. In addition, ENPs have a leadership role in coordinating the MIU team and collaborating with other agencies in 'whole systems working' to address patient journey priorities. Advanced practitioner characteristics: 'understands system', 'visionary', 'creative critical thinker' and 'good interpersonal abilities' are valuable in this respect.

Creative thinking in whole systems and patient journey stages/priorities

As discussed in Chapter 3, whole systems theory refers to the complex organizational context in which healthcare is delivered and the implications for coordinating services effectively to address public health needs and facilitate service user participation (Pratt et al. 2005). NHS principles and values, giving access to free healthcare for all, are applied in the policies and culture of the MIU that provides a 24-hour, seven-days-a-week service. The ability to continuously cope with treating unpredictable numbers and types of injuries depends on good communication and collaboration and shared priorities within a wide network of complementary and interdependent agencies, based in MIUs, hospitals and the community as illustrated in Table 6.3.

Table 6.3 Network of agencies with whom ENP in a nurse-led minor injury unit (MIU) communicates and collaborates to deliver safe and effective care

NETWORK OF AGENCIES WITHIN THE MINOR INJURY UNIT (MIU)
Patient plus relatives and friends accompanying patient.

MIU Personnel: receptionist, triage nurse, healthcare assistant (HCA), ENP

NETWORK OF AGENCIES WITHIN WIDER HOSPITAL ENVIRONMENT
Allied health professionals: radiographers, biochemists, haematologists, pharmacists, physiotherapists

Specialist medical practitioners: accident and emergency (A&E), orthopaedics, ophthalmology, ear, nose and throat, maxillary-facial, obstetrics-gynaecology, genito-urinary, surgery, medicine, paediatrics, elderly care

Managerial, nursing and others: hospital managers, matrons, clinical managers, shift coordinators, bed managers, nurses based in wards/A&E/specialist units, patient transport service, paramedics/ambulance crew

NETWORK OF AGENCIES WITHIN THE COMMUNITY
General practitioners (GPs), dentists, police, social workers, on-call GP service call handlers, GP receptionists, community/district/practice nurses, health visitors, child protection nurses, safeguarding nurses (for vulnerable adults), mental health crisis intervention team, carers in nursing homes and care homes, wardens in sheltered housing, other relatives or friends of patients, patients' employers

Patients and accompanying friends or relatives join with MIU personnel in a departmental network of agencies (Table 6.3) which is involved in all 12 stages and priorities of the patient journey (Table 6.1). The wider hospital network of agencies includes allied health professionals, specialist medical practitioners, and managerial nursing/others who contribute to investigations, diagnosis, and treatment decisions (Stages 6, 8 and 9), and transfer to and from the MIU (stages 1 and 12). The varied network of agencies in the community provides support following discharge from MIU (stage 12).

Every part of this 'whole system' has an important contribution to make in emergency care and no part of the system can function effectively without the support of other parts. A shared commitment to patient-centred collaborative care is the 'glue' needed to unite the system's different elements, for example, the case study involved effective, timely communication and collaboration within and between patient and partner, MIU personnel, hospital, and community agencies.

However, communication problems do occur, especially at night or weekends when ENPs need to contact an agency which, unlike emergency services, does not offer full 24-hour access. Therefore, creative thinking skills (Simpson and Courtneay 2002) are needed by ENPs to be flexible in responding to continuous, often simultaneous challenges, adapting to changing circumstances using available resources to create or revise solutions to problems arising from patients' injuries. ENPs also have opportunities to use creative thinking skills in a more strategic 'whole systems' role as members of multidisciplinary planning teams contributing ideas to the collaborative development and review of policies and procedures in emergency care. ENPs do not simply follow standardized guidelines, they help design them, applying principles of best practice and evidence-based care.

Reflective activity 6.4

This activity is intended to help you relate interprofessional/multi-agency collaboration, integration and networking, associated with whole systems theory, to care priorities in your area of practice.

1. Think of a patient you cared for and write down all the different agencies involved in their care.
2. Describe the contribution to care made by each identified agency/healthcare professional.
3. Describe your contribution and how this affected and was affected by care given by others.
4. Identify your 'patient journey' stages/priorities (Reflective activity 6.1) for steps 2 and 3 above.
5. To what extent did different agencies/healthcare professions have similar or different priorities?
6. Can you identify an example of interprofessional collaboration to develop policies/procedures?
7. How might patient-centred, interprofessional/agency care be enhanced in your practice area?

Collaborative networking between different agencies (Table 6.3) enables existing services to be better coordinated 'whole systems' and this means they function more efficiently in care delivery. However, it is possible for health professionals to work at maximum efficiency and not address all clinical needs if there is an imbalance between supply (structure of services) and demand for them.

The organization and distribution of NHS services should, therefore, reflect the demographic and geographic profile of the local population. NHS reform encourages whole systems working and identifies emergency care as a priority (DH 2001) but this has led to fewer (albeit well-equipped), centralized A&E departments, resulting in additional travel time and possible delays for patients in accessing urgent care. This means more people attending fewer A&E centres making the health target of completing treatment within four hours more difficult to achieve. This impacts on the MIU in the case study (formerly A&E department) as people attend who should go to the designated A&E centre 20 miles away. It is not unusual to have only one ENP on duty and rarely more than two in the MIU dealing with over a hundred patients during a 12-hour night shift. The pace at which staff need to work to meet the four-hour target raises questions about the quality of care provided. Such risks are likely to remain 'invisible' unless an error occurs that requires investigation.

It is ironic that the quality of care could be potentially undermined by hurrying through a long list of patients to comply with a four-hour target that serves as an indicator of good healthcare. It appears unwise to prioritize a four-hour target irrespective of clinical needs (volume of patients and complexity of problems) and organizational capacity (manpower, skill mix, equipment and resources) to meet the target. Nevertheless, such measurable outputs are used as indicators to monitor standards of care via clinical governance (Temple 2000; Freeman 2002) and failing to comply with targets may result in a financial penalty that can exacerbate resource problems in meeting clinical demand. So, in addition to prioritizing serious complaints, all problems, whatever their nature or however many there are, are required to be prioritized in compliance with a maximum treatment time of four hours.

The health target of completing emergency care for each patient within four hours was achieved in the case study. However, it is limited as an indicator of the actual quality of care provided because compliance does not necessarily mean good care and non-compliance does not necessarily mean bad care. Indicators need developing which prioritize patients' experience of treatment and quality of interventions used in interprofessional healthcare, but this takes time. Time is also needed to reflect on practice and for professional development that could enhance the quality of care given.

Reflective activity 6.5

This activity is intended to help you relate government policy/health targets/structure of services, in the context of whole systems theory, to care priorities in your area of clinical practice.

1. Identify health or social policy or legislation that you feel impacts on your area of practice and give examples of how care delivery, and/or management is affected.
2. Identify government health targets and related care priorities that can be applied to your area of practice and reflect on how well you think they truly represent high quality patient care.
3. Describe the quality indicators used to audit standards and achievement of care priorities in your area of practice and reflect on how well you think they truly represent high quality care.
4. Reflect on what you feel are the main priorities of care in your area of clinical practice and write down what you think would make good indicators in observing whether priorities are being met.

5. To what extent does the organizational structure in your area of practice enable effective whole systems working and what improvements might be made to effectively address care priorities?

6. Ask one or two of your colleagues to do steps 1–5 of this activity, compare results, and repeat the process with other colleagues/health professionals, then consider how to apply the findings.

Lifelong learning in clinical decision-making and patient journey stages/priorities

Addressing the stages and priorities of the 'patient journey' (Table 6.1) is a two-way process as practitioners do not simply apply existing knowledge, they also potentially discover new knowledge via individual/ interprofessional interventions with patients. This is inevitable if patient-centred care is applied; every patient is different so practitioners have to continually adapt plans accordingly. So, in the act of caring, practitioners continually learn from patients what it is they need and then apply this knowledge to prioritize specific goals for their individual care. As discussed in Chapter 4, this is a form of informal work-based learning that complements formal university-based learning in developing professional competence (Cheetham and Chivers 2001). It also explains how practitioners gain and apply 'knowing-in-action' (Schön 1987) to practise. So, despite little time for formal educational sessions within the MIU, it is arguably an environment conducive to lifelong learning in clinical decision-making due to an abundance of informal work-based learning opportunities in caring for a high volume and variety of patients. However, knowing what it is you know and explaining it is difficult, due to the tacit nature of both professional knowledge and the process of informal work-based learning, and a lack of time for reflection in the MIU. One way to identify ENP tacit knowledge is to apply a 'PROFESSIONAL' taxonomy of work-based learning.

'PROFESSIONAL' taxonomy (Cheetham and Chivers 2001) of ENP work-based learning

P   **Practice and repetition:** Conducting systematic physical examination, reviewing X-rays

R   **Reflection:** Think about the significance of observations and implications for treatment

O   **Observing and copying:** How to prepare and apply a plaster cast to hand/wrist/forearm

F   **Feedback:** Patient verbal/written evaluation, audit of records, peer support/assessment

E   **Extra-occupational transfer:** Giving first aid at sporting events with St John's Ambulance

S   Stretching activities: Assess/treat high volume/variety of patients under pressure of time

S   Switching perspectives: Understand patient's perception of pain/ restricted hand movement

I   Interaction with coach: Discuss how to explain, analyse, evaluate, and publish care given

O   Osmosis – unconscious absorption: Senses perceive the look and feel of the injured hand

N   Neurological/psychological   devices/techniques: Applying Neighbour's consultation model

A   Articulation: Documenting/explaining care, letters to GP/Fracture clinic, writing chapter

L   Liaison/collaboration: Patient and partner, MIU team, radiographer, orthopaedic surgeon

The above application of Cheetham and Chivers' 'PROFESSIONAL' taxonomy relates different aspects of ENP tacit knowledge used in the case study to each category of work-based learning. It reveals various forms and sources of tacit knowledge and in doing so makes them more explicit so they can be used for reflection, reviewing practice and identifying professional development needs.

For example, in reflecting on the case study (**R** Reflection) I realized that I often conduct physical examinations almost automatically without being fully aware of steps I am taking (**P** Practice and repetition). This creates difficulties in giving an in-depth explanation of the evidence and rationale for clinical decisions needed in writing this chapter (**A** Articulation). I got help from Michael (co-author) in learning how to identify, analyse and evaluate tacit ENP knowledge/skills by applying theoretical perspectives (**I** Interaction with coach). In this sense the 'PROFESSIONAL' taxonomy (Cheetham and Chivers 2001) is an example of one of its categories, **N** 'Neurological/psychological devices/techniques' as it offers a structure to explain the acquisition and application of professional knowledge within clinical decision-making. Collectively, the categories in the 'PROFESSIONAL' taxonomy convey the knowing-in-action/practice (e.g. **S** Stretching activities), depth (e.g. **R** Reflection), and breadth (e.g. **S** Switching perspectives) of ENPs' tacit knowledge and skills. This complements the characteristics of 'pro-activity – taking initiative', 'critical reflection – reflecting on underlying assumptions' and 'creativity – thinking beyond normal viewpoint' needed by practitioners to maximize work-based learning opportunities (Marsick and Watkins 1990). This can be applied to identify and validate tacit knowledge, question practice and revise actions (Kolb 1984; Lam 2000).

Identifying and validating ENPs' tacit professional knowledge can help to understand and evaluate processes of care, quality of clinical decision-making, and its effect on the patient's experience. It offers a more qualitative understanding of evidence-based practice by including practitioners, patients' and other stakeholders' experience of healthcare, in addition to more familiar quantitative, explicit indicators (Rycroft-Malone et al. 2004), for example, the four-hour health target. By articulating such professional knowledge ENPs and other advanced practitioners may be better able to argue for more staff, resources, time for professional development, or review of policies when necessary. Developing and applying ENPs' tacit knowledge through informal work-based learning, therefore, complements explicit theoretical knowledge gained through formal university-based learning, since both are required to inform clinical decision-making that addresses patients' care priorities.

Reflective activity 6.6

This activity is intended to help you relate lifelong learning in clinical decision-making to practice by exploring your pro-activity/critical reflection/creativity (Marsick and Watkins 1990).

1. Pro-activity and taking the initiative: Please identify everyday examples in your clinical practice where you feel confident in applying clinical decision-making skills. Explain how it is that you know what to do in these situations. Then identify an example of a more challenging situation, explain how you learnt to deal with it, and describe the knowledge and skills you applied. Tip: 'PROFESSIONAL' taxonomy categories **P** Practice and repetition, **O** Observing and copying, **S** Stretching activities and **O** Osmosis – unconscious absorption, all involve learning through active involvement so reflect on above (and Chapter 4) examples of these if needed.

2. Critical reflection of underlying assumptions: How do you know that the knowledge you applied in the above situations (step 1) was reliable? What other information would have been useful to you at the time if you had access to it? Why did you decide upon the actions you took? What alternative actions might you have taken? Looking back, do you think the action you took was the best option to address care priorities? How did you evaluate your decisions and actions? Tip: 'PROFESSIONAL' taxonomy categories **R** Reflection, **F** Feedback, **N** Neurological/psychological devices/techniques and **A** Articulation, all involve in-depth learning to analyse, guide, or explain decisions so reflect on above (and Chapter 4) examples of these if needed.

3. Creativity in thinking beyond normal viewpoint: What knowledge, skills and experience, outside of your professional role, do you possess which you find helpful in doing your current job? What examples can you identify where your understanding of healthcare has increased as a result of interprofessional collaboration and/or seeing things from others' point of view? What qualities/skills would your ideal coach/supervisor need to have, and how would this help you? Tip: 'PROFESSIONAL' taxonomy categories **E** Extra-occupational transfer, **S** Switching perspectives, **I** Interaction with coach and **L** Liaison/collaboration, all involve thinking 'outside the box' and breadth of learning so reflect on above (and Chapter 4) examples of these if needed.

Cognitive continuum theory (nine modes) and patient journey stages/priorities

As discussed in Chapter 5, cognitive continuum theory combines intuitive/experiential and analytic/rational decision theories (and respective tacit/explicit knowledge) in a unified theory that matches the different approaches to variations in structure and demands of decision tasks. It offers a framework to develop, guide or evaluate the matching of decision tactics to decision tasks. Table 6.4 maps a revised cognitive continuum – nine modes of practice (Standing 2008) against patient journey stages/priorities (4–12) and ENP clinical decision-making in the case study.

Table 6.4 shows that seven of the nine modes of practice were applied in the case study. The most frequently used modes are reflective and patient/peer-aided followed by system-aided judgement and critical review of experiential and research evidence. For example, system-aided judgement is used in the consultation by applying Neighbour's five task model (discussed earlier), and in the examination by applying a guide to assessing upper limb injuries (Bickley 2007). It guided how I palpated the patient's wrist, hand, fingers, tendons of finger joints and checked for movement (flexion/extension of fingers/wrist), grip, alignment of bones/joints, tenderness and sign of swelling.

Research modes were least frequently used but this is not surprising as the MIU, where the case study took place, is not a clinical research unit. Scientific investigation was needed to confirm the diagnosis and the X-rays were produced by a specialist form of survey research. Surveys give information where individual responses or characteristics can be compared with a larger population and normative values (Parahoo 2006). X-rays of right hand with palm downwards, side of hand and hand-rotated views, as recommended for hand injuries (Chan and Hughes 2005), were taken.

Miss Cartwright's X-rays were, in effect, an anatomical survey of her right hand that provided quantifiable, reliable evidence of a fractured fourth metacarpal. Radiographic evidence, therefore, enabled accurate diagnosis necessary to plan treatment and care management (Hastings 2006).

Previous research studies were also indirectly applied to inform clinical judgement and decision-making through the critical review of experiential and research evidence practice mode. I had read a research article comparing three different cast techniques to treat hand fractures. The casts varied according to how much movement they allowed the fingers. Results showed no significant difference between casts in healing fractures (Tavassoli et al. 2005). I therefore chose a cast that allowed the patient to flex and extend her (taped together) fingers as research indicated it did not compromise bone healing. In addition, it helped to prevent stiffness in the finger joints and promote circulation, and, it was important for Miss Cartwright, a physiotherapist whose livelihood depended on using her hands, to be able to gently exercise her fingers and minimize any loss of strength.

Table 6.4 Patient journey stages/priorities and cognitive continuum – nine modes of practice

NINE MODES OF PRACTICE

STAGE OF PATIENT JOURNEY	Intuitive	Reflective	Patient/ peer-aided	System-aided	Critical review of experiential/ research evidence	Clinical audit/ action	Qualitative	Survey	Experimental
	J U	D G E	M E	N T		R E	S E	A R	C H
4 Consultation	Sense patient's pain and distress	History of a fall when jogging can account for hand pain	Elicit history of hand injury	Five task model (Neighbour 2005)					
5 Examination	A hunch bone in hand is fractured	Swelling, guarded, restricted movement	Ask patient where it hurts	Guide to assess (Bickley 2007)	Unsure of fracture so need to X-ray hand				
6 Investigation			X-ray dept. asked for help		X-ray hand			X-rays of right hand taken	
7 Review investigation		X-rays explain signs and symptoms			X-rays show 4th metacarpal in 3 pieces				
8 Diagnosis		Need to enable 4th metacarpal to reunite		Guide to assess (Bickley 2007)	Closed comminuted fracture 4th metacarpal				

(continued)

Table 6.4 Patient journey stages/priorities and cognitive continuum – nine modes of practice (*Continued*)

STAGE OF PATIENT JOURNEY	Intuitive J U	Reflective D G	Patient/peeraided E M E	System-aided N T	Critical review of experiential/research evidence R E	Clinical audit/action	Qualitative S E	Survey A R	Experimental C H
				NINE MODES OF PRACTICE					
9 Treatment		Metacarpal not grossly misaligned so surgery may not be necessary	Check if cast is best option with surgeon		Immobilize in cast but allow finger movement (Tavassoli et al. 2005)				
10 Health promotion		Check if cast good fit and patient can move fingers	Ask to return if worried about hand	Guide for patient re. care of plaster cast					
11 Documentation		Final check that tasks and priorities addressed	GP note fracture clinic referral	Standard format for record keeping	Right hand is protected so healing can begin	Peer audit of record of care			
12 Discharge			Follow-up care at clinic	Note time re. four-hour target					

Reflective and patient/peer-aided were the most frequently used practice modes as I continually reflected on the nature of the injury and implications for treatment in collaboration with the patient and multidisciplinary team. For example, I judged that surgery was avoidable because the fracture was closed, in the shaft not head or base of fourth metacarpal, so did not involve joints with finger or wrist bones which would be problematic, and there was no major misalignment of the bone that would have required surgical correction (Eglseder et al. 1997). I needed to check my assessment with the orthopaedic surgeon to be sure a cast was the best treatment, and he agreed that it was.

I was, therefore, constantly switching between different modes of practice according to the nature of decision tasks which supports an assumption of cognitive continuum theory (Hammond 1996). The other assumptions were also supported as my thinking ranged from intuition to analysis; most of the time I used a combination of both; variations in decision tasks prompted different modes of practice; and I applied both pattern recognition and functional relations in processing information.

For example, my intuitive judgement attended to the patient's distress, anxiety about hand injury, dishevelled appearance, acute pain, history of injury, her partner's concern, redness, swelling and restricted hand movement. Together these signs and symptoms enabled pattern recognition of a significant hand injury. Analysis of the X-rays provided definitive evidence of a fractured fourth metacarpal in Miss Cartwright's right hand. This clearly demonstrated specific functional relations between the anatomical cause (fractured metacarpal) and physiological effect (pain in right hand).

In Table 6.4, patient journey stages/priorities (4–12) in the case study are used to structure decision tasks that prompted application of the modes of practice by ENP in clinical decision-making. This provides a concise summary of all the key decisions taken by the ENP in the case study. As such, the revised cognitive continuum – nine modes of practice seems a useful tool to illustrate, analyse, explain, evaluate and develop clinical decision-making in nursing and interprofessional healthcare.

Reflective activity 6.7

This activity is intended to help you relate the revised cognitive continuum – nine modes of practice to stages and priorities of the patient journey and clinical decision-making in your area of practice.

1. Keep a diary of all your activities during a single shift then try to match them to the nine modes of practice in the revised cognitive continuum (Table 6.4). What pattern do you notice?
2. What information processing skills do you associate with the modes you use most often? Refer to previous examples of using pattern recognition

and functional relations and try to identify an example of each of these methods of information processing from your clinical experience.

3. Do you think that the nature of patient needs and decision tasks might benefit from you using a different approach sometimes? What other modes of practice do you need to develop further?

4. Refer to Table 6.4 and draw up your own similar grid making adjustments to the patient journey stages/priorities if necessary to suit your particular area of clinical practice.

5. Identify a case study from your clinical practice, describe all the related decision tasks, and then plot them on the grid according to which mode of practice you think they belong to.

6. How does your grid compare to Table 6.4? Is there a similar or different distribution of modes of practice? How might you apply the nine modes of practice to decision tasks, associated with the different stages and priorities of the patient journey, in your future clinical practice?

Summary

The concept of a 'patient journey' was used to identify stages and priorities of care from admission to discharge in a case study of a patient who fell while jogging and fractured a bone in her hand. Clinical decisions and actions taken were analysed by applying the theoretical perspectives from Chapters 1–5 to the different stages and priorities of the patient journey. Prioritizing decision-making was discussed in relation to: government policy and health targets, for example, that a patient's stay in emergency care should not exceed four hours; a matrix model of nurses' perceptions of clinical decision-making skills; personal characteristics ('understands system' and 'risk taker') of advanced practitioners; whole systems working for integrated collaborative interprofessional care; informal work-based lifelong learning as practitioners care for patients; and, cognitive continuum theory – nine modes of practice regarding stages/priorities of the patient journey. The application of theoretical perspectives in discussing the case study helped to articulate tacit knowledge and skills which are difficult to explain, and easily overlooked. A comprehensive range of reflective activities encouraged readers to apply theory to their own practice to help illuminate, explore and explain their tacit knowledge in providing and prioritizing care. Indeed, knowledge gained from analysing clinical decision-making of advanced practitioners in prioritizing patient care could help to generate a more meaningful set of quality indicators to deliver and evaluate safe and effective practice.

Key points

- Health policy identifies strategic priorities/health targets (e.g. emergency care done in four hours) guiding NHS reform/reorganization, aims of healthcare providers, and structure of services.

- The concept of a 'patient journey' is associated with prioritizing patient-centred care regarding access to care, what needs to be done for the patient at each stage, and clinical quality audit.
- A consultation model: connecting/summarizing/handing over/safety netting/and housekeeping (Neighbour 2005) identifies advanced practitioners' priorities in collaborating with patients.
- In emergency care a triage system prioritizes those patients with the greatest clinical need.
- Each individual patient's care is prioritized to relieve suffering, promote healing/full recovery where possible, assess risks/avoid complications, and enable resumption of healthy living.
- In the case study the ENP applied seven out of nine practice modes in the cognitive continuum including 'critical review of experiential/research evidence' in justifying the intervention used.
- Advanced practitioners are in a position to identify and articulate more meaningful quality indicators of patient-centred/individual care than simply complying with health targets conveys.
- Applying decision theory/research to review case studies is helpful to explain actions, identify inconsistencies in health policy and practice, and inform professional development portfolios.

References

Alberti, G. (2007) *Emergency Care Ten Years On: Reforming emergency care*. London: HMSO.

Bickley, L.S. (2007) *Bates' Guide to Physical Examination and History Taking*, 9th edn. New York: Lippincott Williams and Wilkins.

Chan, O. and Hughes, T. (2005) ABC of emergency radiology. *British Medical Journal*, 330(7499): 1073–5.

Cheetham, G. and Chivers, G. (2001) How professionals learn in practice: An investigation of informal learning amongst people working in professions. *Journal of European Industrial Training*, 25: 246–92.

Department of Health (DH) (2001) *Reforming Emergency Care: First steps to a new approach*. London: HMSO.

Department of Health (DH) (2005a) *Commissioning an 18 Week Patient Pathway: Proposed principles and definitions*. London: HMSO.

Department of Health (DH) (2005b) *Modernising Services for Renal Patients*. London: HMSO.

Department of Health (DH) (2005c) *Tackling Cancer: Improving the patient journey*. London: HMSO.

Dimond, B. (2008) *Legal Aspects of Nursing*, 5th edn. Harlow: Pearson Education.

Eglseder, W.A., Juliano, P.J. and Roure, R. (1997) Fractures of the fourth metacarpal. *Journal of Orthopaedic Trauma*, 11: 441–5.

Fletcher, N., Holt, J., Brazier, M. and Harris, J. (1995) *Ethics, Law and Nursing*. Manchester: Manchester University Press.

Freeman, T. (2002) Using performance indicators to improve health care quality in the public sector: A review of the literature. *Health Services Management Research*, 15: 126–37.

Goldsmith, R. and Lumsden, K. (2008) Minor injury and minor illness management, in L. Howatson-Jones and P. Ellis (eds) *Outpatient, Day Surgery and Ambulatory Care.* Oxford: Wiley-Blackwell.

Hammond, K.R. (1996) *Human Judgment and Social Policy: Irreducible uncertainty, inevitable error, unavoidable injustice.* New York: Oxford University Press.

Hastings, A. (2006) Making the diagnosis, in S. Redsell and A. Hastings (eds) *The Good Consultation Guide for Nurses.* Oxford: Radcliffe Publishing.

Kettenbach, G. (2009) *Writing Patient/Client Notes: Ensuring accuracy in documentation,* 4th edn. Philadelphia: F.A. Davis Company.

Kolb, D.A. (1984) *Experiential Learning.* Englewood Cliffs, NJ: Prentice-Hall.

Lam, A. (2000) Tacit knowledge, organizational learning and societal institutions: An integrated framework. *Organizational Studies,* 21: 487–513.

Marsick, V.J. and Watkins, K.E. (1990) *Informal and Incidental Learning in the Workplace.* London: Routledge.

Maude, P. and Hawley, G. (2007) Clients' and patients' rights and protecting the vulnerable, in G. Hawley (ed.) *Ethics in Clinical Practice.* Harlow: Pearson Education.

Moss, B. (2008) *Communication Skills for Health and Social Care.* London: Sage.

Neighbour, R. (2005) *The Inner Consultation,* 2nd edn. Oxford: Radcliffe Medical Press.

Nursing and Midwifery Council (NMC) (2008) *The Code: Standards for conduct, performance and ethics.* London: NMC.

Parahoo, K. (2006) *Nursing Research: Principles, process and issues,* 2nd edn. Houndmills: Palgrave Macmillan.

Pratt, J., Gordon, P., Plampling, D. and Wheatley, M.J. (2005) *Working Whole Systems: Putting theory into practice in organizations,* 2nd edn. Oxford: Radcliffe Medical Press.

Purcell, D. (2003) *Minor Injuries: A clinical guide.* Edinburgh: Churchill Livingstone.

Redsell, S. and Hastings, A. (eds) (2006) *The Good Consultation Guide for Nurses.* Oxford: Radcliffe Medical Press.

Rycroft-Malone, J., Seers, K., Titchen, A. Harvey, G., Kitson, A. and McCormack, B. (2004) What counts as evidence-based practice? *Journal of Advanced Nursing,* 47(1): 81–90.

Schön, D. (1987) *Educating the Reflective Practitioners.* San Francisco: Jossey-Bass.

Shah, N. (2005a) Taking a history: introduction and the presenting complaint. *Student BMJ,* 13: 314–15.

Shah, N. (2005b) Taking a history: conclusion and closure. *Student BMJ,* 13: 353–96.

Simpson, E. and Courtneay, M. (2002) Critical thinking in nursing education: Literature review. *International Journal of Nursing Practice,* 8: 89–98.

Standing, M. (2007) Clinical decision-making skills on the developmental journey from student to Registered Nurse: a longitudinal inquiry. *Journal of Advanced Nursing,* 60(3): 257–69.

Standing, M. (2008) Clinical judgement and decision-making in nursing – nine modes of practice in a revised cognitive continuum. *Journal of Advanced Nursing,* 62(1): 124–34.

Tavassoli, J., Ruland, T., Hogan, J. and Cannon, D. (2005) Three cast technique for the treatment of extra-articular metacarpal fractures. *Journal of Bone and Joint Surgery,* 87: 2196–201.

Temple, M. (2000) New Labour's Third Way: Pragmatism and governance. *British Journal of Politics and International Relations,* 2(3): 302–25.

Tippins, E. and Evans, C. (2007) Introduction to emergency care, in C. Evans and E. Tippins (eds) *The Foundations of Emergency Care.* Maidenhead: McGraw-Hill.

7 Accountability within interprofessional healthcare

Elizabeth Duck

Overview

This chapter discusses practitioner accountability in interprofessional healthcare within the context of clinical judgement and decision-making by an advanced practitioner in radiotherapy based in a clinical oncology department. Knowledge and skills necessary to implement and sustain changes in practice are outlined which challenge traditional role expectations in the National Health Service (NHS) and demand greater individual accountability. A case study in which as a radiographer I had to apply my newly acquired knowledge and skills is outlined. I attempt to reveal challenging issues arising from a medical request to carry out a procedure for a patient which did not appear entirely warranted, how I dealt with the situation, and how reflecting on this contributed to my professional development. Clinical judgement and decision-making in the case study are discussed applying Adair's Five Step Decision-Making Tool (1997) and Standing's Revised Cognitive Continuum (Chapter 5). Analysis of Critical Incidents (Tripp 1993) is also applied in order to reflect on and evaluate the measures used, results obtained, and implications for practice in future situations. The major issues discussed regarding practitioner accountability in interprofessional healthcare are also applicable to those in other health professions, including nursing, and reflective activities are included to help readers relate chapter content to their own particular area of clinical practice.

Objectives

- Appreciate the importance of clinical knowledge and reasoning within professional judgement in enabling recognition of inconsistencies between evidence-based protocols and individual prescribed treatments
- Understand the role of individual practitioners in contributing to effective multi-disciplinary teamwork including challenging colleagues' actions in the interest of patient safety
- Identify how factors such as role accountability and the presence of risk within the Health Service influence decision-making and underline the importance of reflecting on and evaluating all acts and omissions

- Apply models and tools used in this chapter, such as Adair's 5-step approach to decision-making and Standing's revised cognitive continuum, to reflect on clinical situations experienced as a practitioner in one's own area of expertise and accountability

Background

With an ever increasing competitive consumer society, greater accountability is demanded of all professionals including nurses and radiographers, culminating in the introduction of measurable outcomes of care in the form of policies, contracts, guidelines and protocols. This involves linking target setting and practitioners' skill mix to help ensure the highest standards of practice (Fish and Coles 1998: 7). In this climate of change the role of advanced practitioners in healthcare professions allied to medicine has developed where the acquisition of advanced clinical skills and knowledge leads to increased accountability for their clinical judgements and decisions.

In 1920, Professor C.E.A. Winslow at Yale School of Medicine, USA, defined public health as 'the science and art of preventing disease, prolonging life and promoting health through the organized efforts and informed choices of society, organizations, public and private, communities and individuals'. Government healthcare policy is often guided by health specialists' expert judgement of how to serve the public's best interest in protecting the health of the population (Downie and Macnaughton 2000: 110). These policies are then introduced into hospital policy which regulates clinical procedures within departments such as radiotherapy. Radiotherapy relies heavily on clinical protocol-based practices and procedures, which give some room for autonomy within day-to-day working practice. Written protocols ease the many routine day-to-day decisions, but should not be used as a substitute for all judgements in all situations (Benner 1984: 237). Non-routine circumstances demand questioning and informed decisions being taken by the appropriate people, resulting in judgements and decisions being made and documented. Any variance from protocol, such as the repetition of X-ray imaging, requires written justification from a designated medical referrer such as a consultant oncologist (IR(ME])R, DH 2000a). The radiographers' code of practice stipulates a duty of care towards patients accepted for imaging and treatment, where they are accountable for their actions and able to justify their practice. This includes the ability to identify and acknowledge limitations in knowledge and competence within their scope of practice (College of Radiographers (COR) 2004). Judgement in the clinical setting is, in effect, practical wisdom (Aristotle, trans. 1980), the emphasis being on the appropriateness of the judgement and decision made in a given context to achieve a safe and effective outcome for patients.

Historically patients attending a clinical oncology department for radiotherapy treatment of breast cancer were seen by an oncologist who determined the clinical marking of the treatment area. They then reviewed the beam positioning after X-ray imaging and subsequently prescribed the dose plan which radiographers had calculated based on these parameters. However, traditional interprofessional boundaries are often seen to limit the optimal use of skills and experience within clinical oncology, where competency should be the main criterion for undertaking a particular task (Royal College of Radiologists (RCR) 2002). Therapy radiographers have an essential role to play in the implementation of protocol-based radiotherapy care, ensuring patients' treatment is delivered competently and swiftly, by those who have the correct skills, rather than a specific professional background (DH 2000b). It enables more effective whole systems working and interprofessional collaboration in patient-centred care (Chapter 3).

This has required a redesign and streamlining of existing services in order to reduce long waiting times (DH 2000c), including introducing extended role development in radiotherapy over the last four years. By adapting the Dreyfus model of skill acquisition (1987) it has been shown how role expansion has developed a wider focus for radiographers (Eddy 2008), where judgements are made on a bigger picture operating from a deeper understanding of the service as a whole. Greater emphasis has been placed on work-based systems of learning (Chapter 4) and professional development through re-education has created major changes from within clinical oncology departments (DH 2000a). Consequently, professional judgement has been acknowledged as central to clinical practice (Fish and Coles 1998: 44), where an in-depth skill acquisition in judgement and decision-making is essential (Benner 1984: 5), and valued over and above learning to apply latest technology in specific procedures.

Professional profile

Over the past three years I have followed a practical and academic programme of learning and have achieved satisfactory expertise to enable me to lead a radiotherapy clinic myself, making advanced judgements and decisions, underpinned by an understanding of the knowledge behind the practice, as well as the skills necessary to carry it out (Lave and Wenger 1991: 101). Through 'legitimate peripheral participation' I have watched an oncologist practise within the clinic for many years and through 'situated learning' (Chapter 4) have now developed the ability to carry out this practice myself, my growing involvement in practice increasing my understanding (Lave and Wenger 1991: 37). Together with my medical colleagues I am now part of a newly established community of practice, being the first and only therapy radiographer in the department so far to progress along this line of role development. The confidence I have gained in my knowledge and expertise has enhanced my ability to communicate effectively to the patients I offer a service to (Fish and Coles 1998: 29) which, in turn, helps to develop their confidence in my professional role.

Advanced practice in radiotherapy

Oncologists work autonomously, but for radiographers undergoing role development this is a new experience, and it is necessary to understand the system as a whole in order to gain a deeper understanding of a single part (Lifewatch 1995–2008). I have learned to identify and articulate the principles and reasoning on which my professional actions and skills rests (Fish and Coles 1998: 9). This has enabled me to assess the importance of each particular situation and use my judgement accordingly rather than sticking rigidly to a set order of protocols where necessary. This practical 'know how' (Benner 1984: 2) has helped me match decision tactics to the specific demands of decision tasks (Chapter 5), conferring legitimacy to my role and giving me a sense of belonging to the social structure (Lave and Wenger 1991: 92). However, I am also aware of needing to provide additional explanation and practical application of relevant theoretical or 'know that' research-based knowledge to further enhance my professional practice.

My primary objective was to identify what training I needed in order to fulfil my newly created role. As the structure of the NHS is changing, new training needs have been identified and new models of professional education and training have been developed (Nixon 2001). The Royal College of Radiologists (RCR) has encouraged the more traditional roles to cross-professional boundaries, widening opportunities for professional development, and developing written agreed protocols for the skill mix, outlining clear responsibilities for clinical procedures and decisions (RCR 2002).

The role of the radiotherapy advanced practitioner was newly created, and early on I realized that there was very little published material in terms of support and guidance to be found. Most studies on clinical judgement and decision-making in the care of breast cancer patients have focused on the kind of treatment choices made by physicians and on the underlying factors influencing these choices, and much less on the actual clinical judgement process (Salantera et al. 2003). Physicians have been shown to base their clinical judgements on theoretical knowledge, compared to the more personal-based knowledge of non-medical professionals including radiographers and nurses.

Through the development of advanced practice I became more aware of a need to develop a better understanding of the judgements, decision-making processes, and moral or ethical aspects of my day-to-day practice, in order to become responsible and professionally accountable (Fish and Coles 1998: 33). Being forced into the role of decision-maker without having these skills would be an unwelcome responsibility, and could be perceived as a failure of the system and of those in higher authority to support and understand the individual (Benner 1984: 168). However, with the system and skills in place, there is nothing more satisfying than being faced with a mental challenge and overcoming it (Adair 1997: 38); the more you want to do it, the better you will get.

The following case study outlines a challenging, non-routine situation, which did not fall into any of the department's specific clinical protocols, where I had to rely on my professional knowledge and expertise in order to come to an ethically acceptable and medically safe decision.

Case study

A 64-year-old lady attended my pre-treatment radiotherapy clinic in the Oncology Department. She had previously undergone surgery for breast cancer and the tumour was successfully removed. She subsequently had a consultation with the oncologist to discuss the advisability of a course of radiotherapy in order to reduce the risk of recurrence. Informed consent was obtained and a brief outline given of what this treatment would involve. Now at the pre-treatment stage, I needed to draw the clinical treatment borders on the patient's skin, then obtain a computerized tomography (CT) scan in order to visualize these borders with respect to the patient's internal anatomy including breast tissue, heart and lungs. A compilation of all this information would then enable me to position and modify the applied radiation beams to achieve an optimal radiation dose.

In order to initiate radiotherapy the oncologist had completed a treatment request form, an electronic 'Action Sheet', detailing dose and frequency of the radiotherapy required, the specific area to be treated, the categorization of the disease with respect to the urgency of treatment that was to be instigated, as well as authorization for me personally to carry out the procedure in the oncologist's absence. I, therefore, needed to use my knowledge and expertise to justify that this procedure was appropriate before authorizing medical exposure of ionizing radiation in the form of a CT scan (DH 2000a). This involved checking that information from the patient's notes included: a current letter of referral for radiotherapy from the named oncologist; a correctly completed radiotherapy consent form; and, evidence of a positive histology regarding the presence of cancer as well as details on the surgical margins, lymph node involvement, and hormonal status.

I read the patient's notes before she was called through for her pre-scan chat which would include an identity document (ID) check and confirmation of consent. However, when I read the prescribed treatment on the action sheet signed by the oncologist I found it included a request for an extra field to the neck, which was not mentioned on the completed consent form. I rechecked the histology, but could find no clinical justification for using this extra field. I then rechecked all the details, but still could not find any details tallying with this treatment plan request. At this point I told my colleagues that the scan could not be done with the current information I had to hand, and asked to re-schedule the scanning list until I had made my decision on what to do next.

I could see three options open to me, all of which came with their own risks to both the patient and me. The first was to mark the patient for the three-field technique, as requested by the oncologist on the action sheet, including extra permanent skin tattoos on her neck, knowing that the histology did not justify this. Potential risks associated with this decision are that the patient would have a larger area of skin irradiated than actually required and she would have unnecessary, visible, permanent marks on her neck. It would also compromise my clinical judgement to accept what the oncologist appeared to have requested on paper, even though it went against what I believed was correct.

The second option was to presume that the oncologist had made a mistake in filling out the action sheet, and to carry on and ignore the request for the extra field which the histology supported (but the action sheet did not). If indeed the extra field was required, the patient would have to be brought back for another CT scan to include this area, and a variance from protocol would need to be signed by the oncologist to justify this extra ionizing radiation exposure. In this situation, my presumption that the oncologist had made a mistake, without checking with her first, could cause friction in our current interprofessional working relationship.

The third option I could see was to admit that I was in a position where I could not make an accurate evidence-based decision given the facts that I had, and therefore needed to involve the oncologist in further decision-making necessary to identify the patient's correct treatment pathway. This would mean that the patient would have to wait longer for her CT scan causing disruption to the busy clinic for my colleagues to deal with, and I would have to disturb the oncologist in the middle of a clinic at another hospital, as well as risking losing face with my colleagues by being seen as lacking the knowledge and expertise to make up my own mind in such a situation.

My final decision was that I personally believed that the two-field arrangement was the correct course of action, but as I did not have enough information to make that decision, it was necessary to justify this with the oncologist. I presented the case history and all the pertinent facts to her over the phone and she agreed with my judgement that the action sheet was incorrect and that the two fields were adequate, and thanked me for consulting with her before taking any clinical action. I confirmed with my colleagues that the scan had been revised from three to two fields (excluding neck) after checking with the oncologist, explained to the patient that everything was ready for the mark-up and scan, which I then led in the knowledge that this was indeed the correct procedure.

Analysis of clinical judgement and decision-making

Analysing the case study in retrospect I can identify the course of action I followed using Adair's five basic steps (1997):

1. Define the objective
2. Collect relevant information
3. Generate feasible options

4. Make the decision
5. Implement and evaluate.

During each of these steps I made use of knowledge I had acquired from a continuum of different sources during my professional career. This helped me to make sound evidence-based decisions by matching cognitive tactics to patients' needs (Chapter 5). In this time I had to act responsibly, justify my scope of practice and acknowledge my limitations (College of Radiographers (COR) 2004).

First, the objective of the exercise was defined (Adair 1997: 17), which in this case was for me to lead the patient's radiotherapy treatment planning in the absence of the oncologist, while acting within departmental clinical protocol. Routine knowledge of the radiotherapy planning process gained in practice had given me the benefits of becoming specialized in this field (Schön 2003: 56). Expertise gained through past critical reviews of research evidence (Standing 2008) during situated learning and academic studying has also enabled me to acquire an understanding of best practice for radiotherapy techniques that were employed within the department.

In order to carry out this role I had to collect all the relevant information (Adair 1997: 18), and what became apparent at this early stage of the proceedings was that the information presented to me was inconsistent and did not justify the treatment regime requested for this patient. Tacit knowledge I had built up over the last few years working closely with the oncologist made me aware that, due to the absence of information I judged as critically important, it was, therefore, impossible for me to continue planning the patient's treatment. I made an instant intuitive judgement to delay the scan, and informed my colleagues as well as the patient in order to minimize uncertainty and disruption to the busy clinic.

At this time of uncertainty, reflection in action was important as I had to focus on my intuitive understanding behind my actions (Schön 2003: 56) and my ability to make evidence-based judgements in order to arrive at my planned outcome. Recognizing that this was not a routine case, I had to decide what to do next, so I produced a range of feasible options open to me at that time (Adair 1997: 21). My reflective judgement (Standing 2008) helped me weigh up and value probable consequences and outcomes for each option, for both the patient and myself. I had some time to 'stop the clock' for this patient, but still the pressures were there from the busy clinic and I was needed to plan the next patient while reflecting on what action to take for the first. The option to go ahead and mark the patient for the extra field went against my professional judgement. The only justification for it was that I was working to the oncologist's orders, ignoring my ability to work autonomously. Elements of the personal existed here in my professional judgment too (Fish and Coles 1998: 240) as I would not have wanted unnecessary permanent marks had I been the patient. However, if I decided that the oncologist was wrong and had planned without the extra field, I would have been acting against certain medical requests with the presumption that I knew better, risking stepping over the professional line and losing the professional respect of the oncologist. Overall I needed to develop and apply correspondence competence (Standing 2008) by deciding what would be the most practical, relevant and evidence-based action I could take.

Weighing up all the advantages and disadvantages and their possible consequences (Adair 1997: 24), I made my decision not to scan with the information I had. I justified this decision using my system-aided judgement (Standing 2008) by re-examining all the departmental protocols and disease management material to make sure my decision was clear and evidence-based. The role of advanced practitioner has required me to become more directly accountable for my actions (Schön 2003: 297), and I had to behave in a competent and professional manner, both towards the patient and to the oncologist through assessing the perceived risks attached to this decision not to scan (Adair 1997: 25). At this point it would be common practice to seek peer-aided judgement (Standing 2008) to confirm my decision, but I was the only radiographer within the department with the expertise to make these decisions, and so decided to involve the oncologist as my peer before making any more clinical decisions. Any unforeseeable consequences of my actions could also require me to make further decisions at a later date (Adair 1997: 29).

Implementing my decision to involve the oncologist (Adair 1997: 29) came with its own risks, as I was aware that although she accepted and trusted my professional judgement, I would need to demonstrate coherence competence (Standing 2008) in the form of a logical rationale to justify my decision to question her clinical judgment. I knew that before I could mark up and scan the patient at the point of no return (Adair 1997), I needed the oncologist to remove contradictory information, so I had to communicate clearly and convincingly with her over a telephone connection between busy clinics in different hospitals. I tried to present the situation clearly and confidently in order to establish my credibility (Benner 1984: 142) and enable her to make evidence-based judgements based on the information I gave her. To do this I had to have the confidence to cross the boundary between radiographer and oncologist and leave behind long-held assumptions about how others might see me (Fish and Coles 1998: 239) to enable her to regard me as a colleague and an equal.

On consultation with the oncologist she agreed with my decision, acknowledging that there was misleading information, and that I had made the right decision not to scan before involving her. Once the position had been clarified I could then relay to my colleagues that I had all the correct information and was ready to scan the patient. In evaluating my clinical judgement and decision-making during this incident (Adair 1997: 29), I learnt to have more trust in my ability to intuitively grasp when prescribed treatment, based on conflicting information, needs to be queried, clarified and rectified, and to apply this in future similar situations where necessary (Fish and Coles 1998: 267). The whole process also highlighted the current psychological relationship between myself and the oncologist, and how medical hegemony still reflected my need to gain her approval and acceptance, which given time and a growth in experience and self-confidence should decrease.

Reflective activity 7.1

The above case study is based on my work as a radiographer advanced practitioner within an oncology department but the questions and challenges it generates, with respect to decision-making processes and accountability can be applied to other health professionals with similar experiences. For example, consider the following questions to reflect on and analyse your own practice, identifying ways of improving and developing your role within the working environment.

1. Clinical protocols: Identify a specific clinical protocol/guideline/assessment or evaluation tool used in your practice area and list the pros and cons of relying on this device to guide clinical judgement and decision-making from your experience of applying it to patient care.
2. Routine procedures: Select a clinical procedure routinely applied in your practice area, identify potential threats to safe or effective implementation of the procedure, and specify any improvements that are needed to minimize risks and threats to patient safety.
3. Interprofessional role: Select a patient you have cared for, list all the health professionals involved in the patient's care, compare/contrast their respective contributions and identify their areas of individual practitioner accountability for clinical decisions. Reflect on how your clinical judgement/decision-making may have been influenced by other health professionals and, how in turn, you may have also influenced their clinical judgement/decision-making.
4. Critical incident analysis: Identify a situation you have experienced where you used your clinical judgement and decision-making skills. Apply Adair's five basic steps to describe how you progressed through the process of care delivery. Analyse the reasons for the choices you made during clinical judgement and decision-making in each of Adair's five basic steps with reference to the revised cognitive continuum – nine modes of practice (Chapter 5).

Reflection and discussion

As referred to in Chapter 1, accountability for decisions and actions includes a professional and legal obligation to provide safe and effective care to patients. On a practical level this involves being able to explain and justify to patients, peers and others any clinical procedures that are undertaken on behalf of patients. To be able to do this effectively, principles of evidence-based care and/or best practice need to be applied to demonstrate the reasoning behind using certain procedures (coherence competence) and their practical relevance (correspondence competence) in achieving desirable care outcomes for patients (Chapter 5). For example, in the case study I became aware that there was no apparent therapeutic reason for irradiating the patient's neck and such treatment would not, therefore, be in her best interest. It was the recognition of my individual accountability and duty of care that strengthened my resolve not to simply follow the oncologist's request but to question it. In challenging the prescribed treatment I had to apply characteristics associated with advanced practitioners including being knowledgeable, critical thinking skills, and exercising professional autonomy (Chapter 2) acquired through specialized clinical experience.

I have become aware of continually making judgements and decisions within my day-to-day work as a therapy radiographer and that my clinical expertise has been highly influenced by experience in the area of breast cancer (Benner 1984: 179). I have been able to gain a wider knowledge of my field of interest leading the pre-treatment stage of the radiotherapy, becoming familiar with the variations in the treatment preferences of each individual consultant (Coombs and Ersser 2004) in the absence of solid evidence-based medicine. I also understand that there is always a degree of uncertainty within clinical practice, and how valuable non-routine practice is for the development of my future decision-making experiences (Benner 1984: 178). It is also important to acknowledge the incidence of ambiguous circumstances where it may be necessary to make decisions which are not based on hard facts (Van der Schueren 2000) but on the practitioner's best judgement.

Recognizing the presence of uncertainty should be seen as constructive in the continuation of my self-education, not a defensive issue (Schön 2003: 299) indicating failure. In these situations one of the key skills is asking the right questions (Adair 1997: 36), especially when there is pressure to come to a fast decision due to time restrictions and workload within the department. Once I asked certain questions I realized I was outside my acceptable professional boundaries, and was able to manage and coordinate the situation (Coombs and Ersser 2004) until I made another decision, this time to involve the oncologist. It is initially necessary to take time weighing up all available information to aid clinical judgement, allowing the final decision to have a sound basis, although with experience and increased confidence the practitioner will find that this whole process becomes faster and more straightforward (Fish and Coles 1998: 267).

Medical knowledge and decision-making are historically managed by doctors, while allied health professionals are obliged to cooperate in carrying out procedures to assist the diagnosis and/or treatment of patients. A medical model of care encourages a view that allied health professionals are accountable to doctors for the services they provide and this could be exacerbated where their roles are extended to take on previously medical tasks. However, effective whole systems working (Chapter 3) emphasizes that all health professionals are accountable to patients and the need for interprofessional networking and collaboration to provide high standards of care. I developed a good working relationship with the oncologist including a mutual recognition and acceptance of our new roles (Coombs and Ersser 2004) that reduced potential power conflict (Lave and Wenger 1991: 116) and contentiousness when I questioned the reasoning behind certain clinical judgements. Departmental protocols exist as a list of predetermined factors setting standards for the average patient (Benner 1984: 237) as guidance only for prioritization and decision-making, so I had to be able to use value judgements in order to weigh up each situation separately. Once I had made my decision I needed to put across my case clearly and succinctly to the oncologist, confident in the knowledge I held and ability to explain it, having 'learnt to talk' (Lave and Wenger 1991: 109).

Once I had implemented my decision and the correct information had become available to me I could carry out my objective of planning the patient's radiotherapy treatment, with a view to evaluating the whole decision-making process later in light of my experience. I needed to identify when the problem occurred as well as having a clear idea of possible and probable consequences of my actions (Adair 1997: 36) in order to increase my ability to detect similarities with other non-routine situations (Schön 2003: 315), and how I dealt with them. Through reflection and evaluation I could recall the clinical knowledge I had learned over time (Benner 1984: 41), so I did not forget what was influencing my professional actions and interventions by accepting events without stopping to think and learn from them (Fish and Coles 1998: 155). I therefore decided to create a series of critical incidents for all future non-routine cases, documenting my judgement and decision-making processes (Tripp 1993), and I anticipate that through learning from experience it will allow me to explore and question all my actions and assumptions, as well as to comprehend the consequences of my judgements to the patients in my care.

As I progressed in my learning I decided to create a portfolio of critical incidents (Tripp 1993), in an attempt to identify the main causes of what I judged to be significant incidents, and to assess the judgements and decisions I had made in order to improve my understanding of them. I found it unsettling at first to discover a 'near miss' or potential mistake, and I felt at fault in not preventing the error in the first place (Benner 1984: 143) as I always thought that the oncologist's decisions were beyond doubt. Learning is a continual experience. With increasing confidence in my ability to make sound judgements I now enjoy a new level of responsibility, aware that I must consistently question my judgements and re-analyse my decisions (Tripp 1993: 137). My conclusions so far are that there is usually a sound medical reason for an apparently non-routine medical request, which I possibly do not know about, although there will be times when mistakes have been made, and communication poor. This will hopefully decrease as I become more experienced as I am in the best position to safeguard and coordinate the patient's total care (Benner 1984: 143).

Since writing this case study I have become involved with many more non-standard procedures, highlighting to me how important it is to be aware of my judgement and decision-making methods. All of these cases had clinical information which initially did not add up to the technique requested, were not to be found in clinical protocols, and on reflection could have been made simpler through better communication. One case involved too many inconsistencies from both the oncologist and registrar involved in documenting the treatment of choice, leading me to drawing the wrong conclusions. A rare and potentially highly aggressive tumour diagnosis explained the non-protocol treatment of choice in a second example, which I identified and had to research myself before I could justify the procedure requested. A third case highlighted the oncologist's moral and ethical decision-making process where personal experience and expertise ruled out advanced radiotherapy and chemotherapy treatment due to the patient's co-morbidities and general poor health. A fourth case involved a young patient with aggressive localized disease, with a clinical decision to treat as more advanced. I acted as requested, intuitively feeling this to be the correct procedure with respect to the patient's overall status, even after sleeping on it (Adair 1997). Via peer-aided judgement (Standing 2008) with the oncologist the following day, further previously undocumented evidence of her disease status confirmed these decisions were appropriate.

Absorbing new ideas through practical experience, and becoming aware of the importance of reflection and critical analysis through academic study have enabled me to develop and refine my professional judgements and decision-making skills. This has enabled me to become a more reliable and autonomous member of my new community of practice, benefiting the patient pathway and the smooth running of the department. Continuing to develop my role as an advanced practitioner in the Radiotherapy Department has increased my confidence in my ability to make sound judgements and apply critical interpretation through reflection and analysis. Continual reflection on your own actions will reduce the temptation to lapse into a non-critical state of operating during routine procedures, and will hopefully limit the occurrence of unnecessary errors and mistakes. Clinical audit of non-standard cases has further developed my practice in a more analytical cognitive way (Standing 2008), and has inspired me to undertake future qualitative research in an attempt to resolve some of the uncertainties highlighted within my practice. This will be of help to future advanced practitioners travelling along similar routes to role specialization, as well as improving my own understanding of current events. The increase in knowledge and critical thinking of advanced practitioners underpins their professional autonomy and accountability for decisions. This chapter supports Chapter 3 in showing that individual practitioner autonomy and accountability can actually strengthen effective, collaborative, interprofessional healthcare.

Summary

This chapter has highlighted the important role clinical knowledge and reasoning play within professional judgement. I have attempted to illustrate how necessary it is for the advanced practitioner to understand and work within the limits of their judgement and decision-making abilities, through continual reflection and analysis of the level of skills and knowledge achieved. This is necessary in order to maintain specialist knowledge and skills, as well as functioning as a competent and reliable member of the interprofessional health service organization. Various models and tools are available to assist in appraising our clinical judgement and decision-making skills, enabling us to break down situations in order to understand and deal with co-existing issues.

Radiotherapy treatment planning for patients with breast cancer is a specialized role, traditionally lead by an oncologist, but now with a radiographer as lead. Traditional boundaries have moved, and greater accountability has been assumed by the radiographer, as well as an understanding of interprofessional working relationships. It is of great importance to continually evaluate your own actions as well as those of your colleagues, in order to identify any deviation away from protocol which cannot be easily justified. The ability to acknowledge that you cannot make an informed decision with the facts available to you indicates there is a need for shared decision-making, with the need to identify which member of the interprofessional team needs to be involved. Possessing an understanding of how individuals and multidisciplinary teams make professional judgements, it may then possible to question and challenge colleagues' clinical decisions when necessary, in the interest of patient safety. There is always a danger of slipping into over familiarity within routine work. Acquiring greater professional accountability brings a heightened awareness of the risks involved in all clinical decisions we make every day. It is therefore important to be able to justify all actions, as well as be able to reflect and evaluate situations after they have occurred to identify any scope for improvement, should a similar situation reoccur.

Key points

- Advanced practitioners' accountability for clinical decisions and resulting actions includes a professional and legal obligation to provide safe and effective care for patients.
- Health policy/NHS reform led to extending allied health professionals roles, to reduce waiting time e.g. cancer care, making them accountable for what were once solely medical procedures.
- Demonstrating accountability applies coherence competence to explain and justify decisions and correspondence competence to ensure decisions achieve good patient care outcomes.
- Adair's (1997) five steps: define objective; collect relevant information; generate feasible options; make decision; implement/evaluate, are a useful structure to guide or defend clinical decisions.
- Non-routine situations prompt more clinical judgement by advanced practitioners in assessing risks and deciding what to do, and highlight their individual accountability in defending actions.
- Each practitioner is accountable for their decisions in interprofessional healthcare and needs to check and/or challenge any inconsistencies in vital information given by other team members.

References

Adair, J. (1997) *Decision Making and Problem Solving*, London: Chartered Institute of Personnel and Development.

Aristotle (350 BC) *The Nicomachean Ethics*, translated by W.D. Ross (1980) [Online]. Available at: http://classics.mit.edu/Aristotle/nicomachaen.html (accessed March 2008).

Benner, P. (1984) *From Novice to Expert – Excellence and Power in Clinical Nursing Practice*. Menlo Park, CA: Addison-Wesley.

College of Radiographers (COR) (2004) *Statements for Professional Conduct*. London: COR.

Coombs, M. and Ersser, S.J. (2004) Medical hegemony in decision-making – a barrier to interdisciplinary working in intensive care? *Journal of Advanced Nursing*, 46(3): 245–52.

Department of Health (DH) (2000a) *Ionising Radiation (Medical Exposure) Regulations*. London: DH.

Department of Health (DH) (2000b) *Meeting the Challenge: A strategy for the allied health professions*. London: DH.

Department of Health (DH) (2000c) *The NHS Cancer Plan: A plan for investment, a plan for reform*. London: DH.

Downie, R.S. and Macnaughton, J. (2000) *Clinical Judgement: Evidence in practice*. Oxford: Oxford University Press.

Dreyfus H.L. and Dreyfus S.E. (1987) *Mind over Machine: The power of human intuition and expertise in the era of the computer* [Online] Available at: http://w3.msi.vxu.se/~per/CP-web/PBDDSKIL.HTM (accessed February 2008).

Eddy, A. (2008) Advanced practice for therapy radiographers – a discussion paper. *Radiography*, 14: 24–31.

Fish, D. and Coles, C. (1998) *Developing Professional Judgement in Health Care: Learning through the critical appreciation of practice*, 2nd edn. Oxford: Butterworth-Heinemann.

Lave, J. and Wenger, E. (1991) *Situated Peripheral Participation*. Cambridge: Cambridge University Press.

Lifewatch (1995–2008) *Systems thinking* [Online] Available at: http://www.lifewatch-eap.com/poc/view_doc.php?type=docandid=4405andcn=290 (accessed February 2008).

Nixon, S. (2001) Professionalism in radiography, *Radiography*, 7: 31–5.

Royal College of Radiologists (RCR) (2002) *Breaking the Mould: Roles, responsibilities and skills mix in departments of clinical oncology*. London: RCR.

Salantera, S. et al. (2003) Clinical judgement and information seeking by nurses and physicians working with cancer patients, *Psycho-Oncology*, 12: 280–90.

Schön, D.A. (2003) *The Reflective Practitioner: How professionals think in action*, 2nd edn. Aldershot: Ashgate Publishing.

Standing, M. (2008) Clinical judgement and decision making in nursing – nine modes of practice in a revised cognitive continuum, *Journal of Advanced Nursing*, 62(1): 124–34.

Tripp, D. (1993) *Critical Incidents in Teaching: Developing professional judgement*. London: Routledge.

Van der Schueren, E. (2000) Factors in decision making in the treatment of breast cancer. *Radiotherapy and Oncology*, 55: 205–16.

Winslow, C.E.F. (1920) [Online] Available at: http://www.clintoncountygov.com/Departments/Health/print_page/aboutus.pdf (accessed March 2008).

8 | Short- and long-term risk assessment and management

Douglas MacInnes

Overview

This chapter will examine clinical judgement/decision-making associated with short- and long-term risk assessment and management of potentially aggressive behaviour, in the context of forensic mental health care. Initially there will be a brief description of the main features of this clinical area in providing a secure and therapeutic environment to prevent, contain and modify behaviour which may be harmful to others and/or self. Two case studies are presented to compare and contrast short- and long-term risk assessment and management strategies, used by mental health nurses in secure forensic care. These are analysed and discussed in relation to ten perceptions of clinical decision-making identified in the matrix model (Chapter 1). Reflective activities are included to enable readers to relate risk assessment and management of behaviour to their clinical practice.

Objectives

- Appreciate that injuries to self and others may sometimes be intentionally inflicted
- Awareness of different levels of aggressive, abusive, threatening or violent behaviour
- Understand environmental, relational and procedural security issues in healthcare settings
- Compare/contrast decision-making in short- and long-term risk assessment/management
- Apply the matrix model in analysing and explaining risk assessment/management decisions
- Relate risk assessment and management of behaviour to one's own area of clinical practice

Forensic mental health care

Forensic mental health care is defined by Faulk (2000) as the interface between the criminal justice system and psychiatry. The overwhelming majority of service users have both a criminal history and a formal diagnosis of mental illness, including severe mental health problems such as schizophrenia, bipolar disorder, or personality disorder, and often a secondary diagnosis of substance misuse. Kennedy (2002) states that forensic mental health care differs from other mental health services by including subsystems that are at much higher levels of security than usually necessary elsewhere. Although the main orientation is towards risk awareness and risk management, forensic psychiatry remains an integral part of mental health services for the populations they serve. Care is provided in NHS in-patient or community settings, private hospitals, and penal institutions. The Department of Health (2007a) acknowledges that service users include difficult, dangerous and/or extremely vulnerable people whose behaviours present a risk to themselves as well as others. They can be difficult to engage in assessment, treatment or research. Authors have recognized the need for staff to meet the therapeutic needs of service users while also addressing legal, security and public safety issues. Swinton and Boyd (1999) stated that forensic mental health nurses provide care, control, custody and therapy. They further noted that one of the main challenges in caring for service users in secure units is to respect those who have little respect for others, and who are often aggressive, deceitful, and show little remorse for the consequences of their actions.

This chapter focuses on forensic mental health nursing in secure in-patient hospital settings. Low, medium and high security types of care are available (Scottish Forensic Network 2007 – See Appendix 8.1). Pierzchniak et al. (1999) rated 176 service users in a range of settings and specified criteria in relation to the level of violence presented and perceived level of dangerousness. This guided the level of security required by service users on admission to hospital and has been put into a table format by Kennedy (2002). The level of violence at presentation is noted in Table 8.1.

The perceived dangerousness of behaviour is recorded in Table 8.2. This table also includes the criteria used to guide admission to open wards and forensic

Table 8.1 Violence at presentation as a guide to security needed at the time of admission (Kennedy 2002: 438)

Graveness of violence	Behaviour
High (Grade 1)	Homicide. Stabbing penetrates body cavity. Fractures skull. Strangulation. Serial penetrative sexual assaults. Kidnapping. Torture. Poisoning.
Medium (Grade 2)	Use of weapons to injure. Arson. Causes concussion. Fractures long bones. Sexual assault. Stalking with threat to kill.
Low (Grade 3)	Repetitive assaults causing bruising. Self-harm or attempted suicide that cannot be prevented by two-to-one nursing in open conditions.

Table 8.2 Dangerousness as a guide to security needed on admission (Kennedy 2002)

Admission guidelines	Forensic community services	Open ward/24-hr care	Low secure	Medium secure	High secure
Violence (Grades defined in Table 8.1)	No recent violence	Self-harm Lesser degrees of violence	Grade 3 Public order/nuisance offending	Grade 2	Grade 1
Immediacy	Does not need daily monitoring	Confides in staff	Acute illness or crisis likely to resolve in 3–6 months	Relapses abrupt Unpredictable	Unpredictable Inaccessible to staff
Specialist forensic need	Self-medicates Previous admissions to medium or high secure units Reintegrating with local services	Cannot cooperate with voluntary treatment Compliant when formally detained	Recall or crisis of former medium-high-security patient Current mental state associated with violence	Arson Jealousy Resentful stalking Exceeds low secure capacity	Sadistic paraphilias (psychosexual disorders associated with violence) Exceeds medium security
Absconding	Will not break off contact	If absconded would not present an immediate danger	Impulsive absconding	Pre-sentence serious charge Other obvious motivation to abscond	Can coordinate outside help Past absconding from medium/high security

169

community services as well as low, medium and high secure settings. It can be seen that the grade of violence, the immediacy of the risk posed, the absconding risk and the specialist forensic need are all related to the overall risk posed by an individual and the level of security required upon admission.

In examining key elements contributing to security within forensic mental healthcare settings Kennedy (2002) identifies environmental, relational, and procedural characteristics, as follows:

- **Environmental security** relates to the design and maintenance of the buildings in providing a safe and secure setting that enables containment, observation, treatment and rehabilitation.
- **Relational security** relates to the staff–patient ratio and the amount of time spent in face-to-face contact as well as the therapeutic rapport that is established between staff and service users.
- **Procedural security** relates to the policies, procedures and practices in place for controlling risk. This includes the policies relating to the service user, members of staff, and also the institution.

Kennedy draws the following conclusion based on an overview of the three security elements.

Mental health services maintain a safe and effective process of treatment and rehabilitation through the stratification of patients according to the risks they present. Awareness of the therapeutic importance of environmental, relational and procedural security is valuable in drafting safe treatment plans for patients and in the organization and management of all mental health services. Relational security is by far the most important element in the maintenance of the therapeutic progress of patients.

(Kennedy 2002: 442)

Mental health nurses are the professional group with the most face-to-face contact with service users. Kennedy's conclusion indicates that the decisions made by nurses when interacting with service users play a central part in the treatment process in forensic mental health care settings

Reflective activity 8.1

While forensic mental health represents a highly specialized form of risk assessment/management and care, aggressive behaviour can occur throughout the NHS and so some of the principles may be transferable. This activity is intended to help you to reflect on security in your area of practice.

1. Identify an example of verbal and/or physical aggression you have witnessed in practice and described what happened, what triggered it, who was involved, how it was managed, and your feelings about it both during the event and after it had passed.

2. How might environmental, relational and procedural security (Kennedy 2002) be enhanced to prevent and/or manage such incidents more effectively in your area of clinical practice?
3. What are the qualities and interpersonal skills that you have noticed in someone who is good at diffusing potentially aggressive situations and able to maintain dialogue with those concerned?

Nursing and forensic mental health care

The ward nurse in a secure setting works in a locked in-patient environment and it is likely that the service user is formally detained under mental health legislation and is not able to leave unless permission is granted by the clinical team and in some cases by the Ministry of Justice as well. The impact of serious mental health problems for the user is that these are likely to be distressing and impinge on their ability to function on a day-to-day level. There is a probability they have exhibited levels of behavioural disturbance such as violence to themselves and/or others. Additionally, it is likely they will have had contact with the criminal justice system. Although the user may have been aware of some psychological difficulties, they may not have viewed them as related to their mental health and would not have sought to be admitted to a secure environment. Therefore, there is often the potential for conflict between the user's wishes to be independent and the requirements under the law to formally care for the person in a locked environment. The nurse will also work with the user on a longer-term basis as it is likely that the service will care for the user for a number of years. The service user is likely to have many complex needs (psychiatric, social, financial and behavioural) and these are assessed and intervened upon on a long-term basis. One particular problem for nurses has been discussed by Bowers (2002) who noted that whereas the threat of violence was viewed as external to the role of the multi-disciplinary team, it was viewed as part of the day-to-day role of nurses. One of the main reasons that influenced this difference in the attitudes and experiences of violence was due to the fact that nurses would continually drop in and out of different roles such as being a 'psychotherapist' at one point in time and then having to be involved in the physical restraint of a service user. The fact that nurses would be the main professional group involved in the custody and control of service users made the likelihood of being involved in a violent event more likely.

Chaloner (2000a) wrote about the difficulties in clearly stating the defining characteristics of forensic mental health nursing, concluding that there are five overriding characteristics. These are:

1. Ongoing contact with mentally disordered offenders (not necessarily in secure settings)

2. Working as part of (or in close collaboration with) a dedicated forensic mental health service
3. Development of and participation in nurse-specific activities intended to contribute to the care and management of mentally disordered offenders
4. The ability to differentiate between the social and therapeutic aspects of the forensic mental health nursing role and to practise effectively with regards to both
5. An understanding and acknowledgement of the contribution that personal attributes and values make to forensic mental health care.

Chaloner's characteristics complement and can be combined with the UKCC's (1999) examination of nursing in secure environments describing specific areas of nursing competency when working in forensic settings. These areas of competency are: safety and security; assessment and management of risk; management of violence and aggression; therapies; knowledge of offending behaviour and legislation; report writing; and practical skills such as first aid.

Two case studies will be presented to illustrate this area of practice. They examine the clinical decisions made by nurses in relation to assessing and managing risk which is an important element of the nurse's role in secure settings. Case study 1 examines the responses to a short-term and immediate risk situation while Case study 2 examines a longer-term assessment of risk and its associated management strategy. The matrix model (Chapter 1) is applied to analyse decisions made by the nurses using the ten perceptions of clinical decision-making skills as a template for the discussion. It is acknowledged that many decision-making characteristics are not unique to one category but their placement in the matrix is appropriate for the decisions referred to, and it illustrates the many features of decision-making in forensic mental health care settings. Tables 8.3 and 8.4 summarize perceptions of clinical decision-making and conceptions of nursing in a matrix model that represents each case study, respectively.

Professional profile

The author has had 25 years experience of working in forensic mental health settings including working as a nurse in forensic mental health wards and as a researcher in forensic and prison settings. He is joint facilitator of the UK Mental Health Research Network (MHRN) clinical research group; member of Service Users and Carers Experiences of Secure Services (SUCESS), and is also a member of the Royal College of Psychiatrists working group looking into the management of violence. The cases studies described are based on real clinical situations encountered during the author's experiences as a clinician and researcher. Some of the personal details have been changed to preserve the confidentiality of the individual service users. The situations chosen reflect those regularly faced by nurses in forensic mental health care settings.

Case study 1

John is a young male aged 22 who was admitted three months ago to a low secure ward under Section 3 of the Mental Health Act. He was admitted with a diagnosis of borderline personality disorder and has long history of alcohol and illegal substance abuse. He has had a number of short-term admissions to acute mental health wards where he has frequently been abusive, confrontational and disengaged from staff. In the community, he is frequently abusive and violent towards other members of his family and threatening towards other people especially after having drunk alcohol. Since his admission to the ward, John has often been verbally abusive and threatening and there have been repeated attempts to leave the ward without permission. These confrontations have resulted in a number of circumstances where the nursing staff have intervened using physical restraint to resolve the situation. No leave outside the unit has been granted. There has been one incident of a physical assault on a fellow service user which occurred after John had been drinking (after alcohol had been clandestinely brought onto the unit). One weekend, staff members are confronted by John who is in an agitated state and is demanding that he be allowed to leave the unit to visit his sick mother. He is threatening in his manner and states that he will 'hurt someone' unless his request is granted. The decision that staff members have to make is how to respond to this request.

Analysis of Case study 1 (cs1)

Since the clinical team had not agreed that John should have leave (especially outside the hospital), the nursing staff would not be in a position to agree to the request, and as it was the weekend, it is unlikely other members of the multi-disciplinary team would be available to consult. The decision-making process that the nursing staff will follow relates to the view that this specific incident is short term. The immediate ways of dealing with the request and John's agitation are to ensure the situation is managed in as relaxed and non-threatening way as possible, as well as giving potential pointers to managing John in the longer term. The decisions and interventions used by nurses are directed by the guidelines on dealing with immediate and short-term violence/risk (Royal College of Psychiatrists 1998; NICE 2005).

Collaborative decision-making (cs1)

When being confronted with a service user in an agitated state, it is imperative that all members of the clinical team are aware of the situation. This allows a coordinated response from staff to be implemented as well as allowing staff to manage the wider ward environment (NICE 2005) through either informing other service users about what was happening with John (in a general way to avoid breaching confidentiality) or to ensure the physical environment is safe and non-threatening. Usually, this would involve one or two staff discussing the request with the service user face to face in a communal area or within a room where there was some privacy for the user but which could be easily observed and was accessible by other nursing staff. The staff need to discuss options, agree a strategy for managing the incident, and be suitably deployed in speaking to John or in ensuring the safety of others while monitoring the progress of colleagues with John.

Experience and intuition in decision-making (cs1)

It is important that nursing staff are aware, and have previous knowledge and experience, of John's behavioural patterns and the potential areas of flashpoint. This is vital to be able to make a clear decision about the response to the demanding behaviours. As Scott (1977) noted, the best predictor of future behaviour is past behaviour. If it was known that certain behavioural actions were predictive of an escalation in John's level of aggression (and potentially related to the likelihood of an imminent act of aggression) or that he was unlikely to assault others unless he was under the influence of alcohol, this would allow staff to decide whether to allow John to continue to be verbally abusive or whether a formal nursing intervention might be required. Experience of the situation would also be helpful for the nurse(s) who might be subject to the verbal abuse. It is a difficult situation for someone to be in with an agitated person shouting at them and making quite major threats to their safety (irrespective of the likelihood that person may or may not physically assault them). If they had experienced verbal abuse directly or indirectly through observations, it could well reduce the negative impact of being faced with John's verbal abuse (Nolan et al. 1999).

Reflective activity 8.2

What, in your experience, can help you to understand and cope with potentially aggressive or abusive behaviour of patients/others without taking it personally or reacting aggressively yourself?

Confidence in decision-making (cs1)

It is an important feature of the nurses' decision-making that they are able to have confidence in their ability to handle this situation with John to be able to calm him down and minimize the threat to him, staff and service users. Research has shown that the perceptions of the ward environment can dictate how service users view the ward and the consequent levels of disturbance on the ward. If a ward is perceived as unsafe by service users, they are more likely to have increased levels of anxiety, delusional activities and are more likely to be involved in disturbances (Quirk et al. 2004). When staff members are perceived as confident and capable in responding effectively when in this situation, it is likely that other service users will feel safe in the ward environment.

Reflective activity 8.3

If practitioner confidence is associated with a calming or reassuring effect upon patients then a lack of it or indeed over-confidence might stimulate anxiety and a potentially aggressive reaction. What helps you to strike the right balance in feeling and demonstrating confidence in your practice?

Systematic decision-making (cs1)

The approach used will vary. It is often the case that taking someone to a quiet area will reduce the level of agitation. Similarly, getting them to sit down in a chair and talk to an attentive member of staff member who responds in a calm manner can also be helpful in reducing agitation. Research has shown that once an agitated service user is able to start to engage in conversation this reduces the level of disturbance and the likelihood of physical assault (Whittington and Wykes 1996). It may also be helpful to allow John to discuss the specific circumstances that had arisen for him to make his request to see his mother, and to offer alternative suggestions such as offering to ring the hospital or a family member to get an update about her condition or enable John to do this.

Prioritizing decision-making (cs1)

The nursing staff will need to ensure that the safety and security of the ward are not compromised so that all people (staff, service users, visitors) are not put at risk. Although the nurses will be aware that when someone is abusive and threatening in a communal environment this can be distressing for on-lookers, this will be balanced against the distress that may be caused if the nurses take a more direct approach. If the view is that the agitation being displayed by John does not constitute a threat to safety then the nursing staff will allow the situation to continue with the approach being to allow John to ventilate his feelings. However, if it is thought that the safety of the ward is beginning to be compromised, for instance, John's behaviour escalates from verbal abusive to displaying violent behaviour towards inanimate objects like throwing chairs against a wall, then the priority may change to ensure the safety and well-being of people on the ward, and some form of intervention such as asking John to take time-out in his room will be required. Prioritizing will also be used when determining the numbers of staff required that should remain on the unit. The numbers judged to be required are those viewed as appropriate to deal with any difficulties. This may mean that other service users might need to be talked to about postponing any escorted leave.

It may also be necessary to prioritize which staff members are deployed to speak to John. Certain staff may be able to generate a more relaxed interaction with John (such as a key worker or a nurse that John has a good relationship with) or there may be some attributes that John is known to like or dislike and these may impact on John's mood and behaviour with nursing staff. Therefore issues such as gender, age, and ethnicity might need to be borne in mind when deciding which nurses should be involved in discussions with John (Royal College of Psychiatrists 1998).

Reflective activity 8.4

Do you think that you are absolved of your duty of care to patients if they become verbally abusive, threatening, or physically aggressive to you or others? If not, what would you do to encourage them to calm down? At what point would you decide that alternative measures are needed?

Observation in decision-making (cs1)

During the period that staff are in close proximity with John they will be closely observing his verbal and non-verbal behaviour to ascertain whether there have been any changes in his demeanour during discussions with him following his request for leave. Any change will be noted and decisions about further interventions will be based upon this evidence. If John is gradually becoming more amenable to discourse and less tense in his body posture, the nurses are likely to continue with their discussions with him and might ask if he would like to discuss his concerns in an area with more privacy. It may also mean that the number of staff needed in the immediate area can be reduced as the likelihood of an aggressive incident is reduced. Although the situation may have become more relaxed, nurses will continue to monitor and record John's behaviour over the rest of the shift (and beyond) to ensure that the agitation does not reoccur and to record the impact of the response to John's agitation over the longer period. Vinestock (1996) described the importance of this, suggesting that the recording of comprehensive reliable information is the central focus of any assessment of risk. In addition, staff will also be monitoring the situation on the rest of the ward. It may be the case that John's outbursts have caused irritation among other service users or they may have sympathy for his request and are irritated with staff for their perceived intransigence. Observations on other service users (and visitors) will guide nurses as to whether any additional intervention is required to ease any disquiet among them or their visitors.

Standardized decision-making (cs1)

The management of violence and aggression has been widely reviewed over the past 40 years and there are numerous guidelines for nurses to use to identify the likelihood of imminent violence and evaluate a range of options with regard to potential interventions. Although these might not always be easily remembered or recognized at the time (especially for nurses new to this specialist area of mental health), they give a good overview of what should be considered. Current national guidelines give clear advice on assessing, evaluating and intervening when someone with mental health problems is acting in an aggressive manner (NICE 2005). Decisions regarding use of de-escalation techniques, time-out, control and restraint, medication, and rapid tranquillization are all discussed. The focus is on intervening in a range of scenarios and the guidelines act as a useful resource for examining different potential interventions and their efficacy in particular situations. There may also be local NHS trust guidance (usually based on national guidelines) for members of staff to follow when dealing with incidents like John's situation. Although nurses may choose a different approach, they need to be aware that they could be required to justify not adopting the intervention detailed in the local guidelines if any untoward occurrence arises from the incident.

Although John has only been in the unit for three months, there has already been one incident within the unit and several episodes of verbal abuse as well as a history of physically assaulting others. The clinical team would be aware of this and would have included this in their overall risk assessment and risk management plan. It is probable that the care plan would include guidelines for dealing with John when he becomes disturbed and that all nurses would be aware of this plan. This care plan would also be guided by the national and local clinical guidelines noted above.

Reflective activity 8.5

What national and local guidelines regarding the prevention and management of aggressive or violent behaviour are recommended for use by your NHS trust or other employing authority? How familiar are you with your rights and responsibilities if confronted by aggressive patients or others?

Reflective decision-making (cs1)

The immediacy of the situation reduces the ability of nursing staff to be able to reflect much upon what has been happening with John while the atmosphere remains tense and difficult. It is only when the incident has been resolved and no further disturbance is foreseen that nurses are able to reflect upon the episode and their role in it. The use of critical incident reviews is recommended by NICE (2005). The reflection can take different forms with some reflection devoted to the emotional response of being threatened or abused and how the nurse has viewed this. The responses to the behaviours exhibited by John will also be reflected on (usually in collaboration with other members of the clinical team) and then recorded with specific emphasis on any contributory factors that may have played a part in the onset of the agitated behaviour as well as those factors (including nursing interventions) which may have heightened or reduced the level of agitation. It is also likely that John's key worker would approach him within a couple of days following the episode to ask him for his views as to what happened and the reasons for his agitated outburst. This process of getting evidence from John, nursing staff and any other persons involved gives information in relation to how and why John acted in the way he did and what helped, or did not help, improve the situation. The inferences drawn from these discussions should be written down to allow other members of the clinical team to be aware of the event and the way in which it unfolded. These conclusions can also be discussed at John's next clinical review with all members of the clinical team involved in John's care. The conclusions drawn might also act as a basis for planning future care such as anger management training, social skills training, medication change or developing closer family ties and increasing visits from John's family. These future interventions would be seen as helping John become less agitated and reducing the likelihood of a similar situation arising again or helping to develop strategies to alleviate his agitation if a situation did arise.

Ethical sensitivity in decision-making (cs1)

The main element of ethical sensitivity revolves around the need to ensure that John is treated fairly both during the course of discussions with staff and also following the incident. It may be that nurses could feel alienated from John (especially if they have been subject to threats and abuse) but there is a professional requirement to ensure that all service users are able to access the best possible care and that the care administered by nurses is equitable to all users (NMC 2008). At times, a senior nurse may be involved in supervision with junior staff and the above issues can be discussed in a safe and supportive environment. Nurses also need to ensure that no personal information should be discussed by nurses about John or his family to anyone not directly involved in John's care and treatment. At times, nurses may feel the need to talk about their experience or stress at work before being able to relax. Although, it may be helpful for nurses to 'offload' in this way to a friend or family member, it is essential that this is done without describing any formal information about John that could identify him as the individual involved (NMC 2008).

Reflective activity 8.6

How might breaching patient confidentiality exacerbate aggressive behaviour in your clinical area?

Accountability in decision-making (cs1)

All of the decisions made by nurses are underpinned by the NMC Code (2008), which notes that nurses are personally accountable for actions and omissions in practice and must always be able to justify decisions made. The nurses on the ward are accountable for the safety and security of all the people on the ward and to ensure that no-one in their care jeopardizes the safety and security of the wider community. In addition, nurses in this situation are under a legal obligation to ensure that the restrictions John is subject to under the Mental Health Act 1983 are adhered to by the team. This would mean that unless there are extremely unusual circumstances, such as the safety of the ward was seriously undermined, John would not be allowed outside the hospital. The nurses are also accountable for the well-being of the other service users on the ward. It may therefore mean that if the situation is unresolved after a period of time and the situation on the ward remains tense, the nursing staff may need to request that additional staff be employed on the ward to allow a more focused approach to be undertaken with John. This would allow activities, intervention and support to be available for other service users on the ward as well. A decision-making matrix indicating the pattern of nurses' responses to John is shown in Table 8.3.

Case study 2

André is a 52-year-old man currently residing in a medium secure unit having been admitted two years previously from a high secure hospital under Section 37/41 of the Mental Health Act. Following the terms of the legislation that André was admitted to hospital under, the Ministry of Justice has to agree to any relaxation of the security arrangements regarding André's care. He has been an in-patient in the high secure hospital for over ten years following a multiple homicide which occurred when he had paranoid delusions concerning the neighbours in the flat above. He lit a fire in the upstairs hallway and the neighbours died as a result of the fire. This included a young child. The incident was reported nationally and there is still local interest in the case. He has been treated successfully on antipsychotic medication and there have been no recorded behavioural management or psychiatric problems since the commencement of treatment soon after his admission. He has been allowed out in the grounds of the medium secure unit without any nursing escort for the last six months and there have been no recorded concerns. He has now requested to be allowed on escorted leave outside the hospital as part of his continuing rehabilitation programme. The decision to be made is whether escorted leave should be given to André.

Analysis of Case study 2 (cs2)

The assessment of risk and decision in response to André's request is of a longer-term nature than John's situation in the previous case study. Therefore more time is available to implement a robust and systematic decision-making process that enables the most efficacious judgment. The decision-making process described in this case study is guided by recommendations for assessing and managing risk documented by the Department of Health (2007b).

Table 8.3 Matrix of decisions made in relation to Case study 1

	PERCEPTIONS OF CLINICAL DECISION-MAKING									
CONCEPTIONS OF NURSING	Collaborative	Experience & Intuition	Confidence	Systematic	Prioritizing	Observation	Standardized	Reflective	Ethical Sensitivity	Accountability
Caring										
Listening & being there										
Practical procedures										
Knowledge & understanding										
Communicating										
Patience										
Teamwork										
Paperwork										
Empathizing & nonjudgemental										
Professional										

Collaborative decision-making (cs2)

Deciding whether André is allowed to have escorted leave is a collaborative decision. MacInnes (2000) stated that it was imperative to get objective and comprehensive accounts from as many sources as possible of any incidents that might inform the risk assessment process. Therefore, the decision regarding André's request involves all members of the multidisciplinary team operating in a democratic manner. It also involves the service user and their carer in this collaborative decision-making process (DH 2007b). Within the unit there will be clear guidelines and procedures for discussing André's request and the roles of each member of the clinical team in terms of gaining relevant information and their role in the final decision. Initially the reasons for the request will be discussed between André and his key worker and it may also be useful to discuss the request with other family members if André has a positive relationship with them. Members of the clinical team involved in André's care will be involved in making a recommendation to the Ministry of Justice if they perceive that the request is something that is reasonable at this point in time. The discussions take place at the ward review and will involve all members of the team giving their views of André's progress thus far and their perceptions as to the correctness or not of the proposed escorted leave. Any concerns or objections would be raised. The nursing staff would most likely have had the majority of contact with André and so their report on his behaviour, mental state and level of risk would be an important part of the discussion. Nurses are the professional group who would provide any escort and therefore any particular concerns or requests for feedback from other members of the clinical team would be noted at this meeting. If agreed by the team, the consultant psychiatrist (as the professional legally responsible for André's care) would write to the Ministry of Justice requesting a specified relaxation of the restrictions imposed upon André.

Reflective activity 8.7

Identify the roles that different colleagues play within multidisciplinary clinical decision-making in relation to risk assessment and management of aggressive behaviour in your area of practice.

Experience and intuition in decision-making (cs2)

One of the main ways that nurses would form an opinion about the appropriateness of this request would be through their experience of assessing risk in forensic mental health care and experience of interacting and working with André (Holloway 1998). It is usual that prior to the Ministry of Justice agreeing for someone to be allowed escorted leave, the service user had received a significant period of in-patient treatment. This period would have allowed the nursing staff to build up a therapeutic relationship with André and to make informed judgements about his mental state, his behaviour and the appropriateness of him being granted escorted leave at that moment in time. They would also have access to his records from the High Secure Hospital and this would allow an assessment to be made of his progress, and any contraindications for supporting the request.

Confidence in decision-making (cs2)

The nursing team must feel confident about being able to give a clear and accurate reflection of how André has been when on the ward since his admission and some assessment of his mental state, his level of engagement, his reaction to being challenged, and his capacity to cope with any disappointments. There would also be an examination of his views about the fire setting but also the relationship between his mental state and the criminal act and whether he was aware of the factors that might indicate that his mental state was deteriorating. Experience in working with people in forensic settings gives nurses a good grasp of these issues and this will guide whether they think the request is worth supporting or whether they have any concerns about the patient's state of mind or potential for violent behaviour. Guidelines are also in place that state that nurses should receive updated risk assessment and risk management training every three years to help in the development of their competence in making judgements about risk (DH 2007b).

Systematic decision-making (cs2)

All elements of the process for assessing André's request and the risk management strategy will be based on the recognition that there are positive aspects to André's individual character and that the principle of recovery from mental illness underpins all rehabilitative approaches in mental health care (Mueser et al. 2004). The request for escorted leave will be part of a phased discharge strategy that would have started when André was admitted to the high secure hospital (Reed 1992). A therapeutic mixture of interventions including medication, psychological therapies, group work, day-to-day contact and observation of behaviour is the cornerstone of treatment, and monitoring André's response to this may enable gradual reduction in the level of restrictions faced.

Reflective activity 8.8

Describe how risk assessment and management are applied in relation to discharge planning and aftercare arrangements for patients/clients/service users in your area of clinical practice.

Prioritizing decision-making (cs2)

Prioritizing focuses on ensuring that care is balanced against any security concerns that may have arisen. It is acknowledged that not all risk can be foreseen. However, it is part of the expertise of nurses in this area that, within the framework of a carefully constructed risk management strategy, positive risk management will be undertaken. In André's case, this means judging whether relaxing his security will be able to happen without any untoward incident happening. Underpinning this positive risk management is the ability of nurses to identify and evaluate the potential risks that André may pose and to be able to make judgements on the likelihood of these actually occurring, and ways in which such risks can be minimized or negated (Tennant *et al.* 2000).

Observation in decision-making (cs2)

Good observation is fundamental to any well-judged risk assessment and also in determining the most appropriate risk management strategy (DH 2007b). Nursing staff would be observing closely any changes in mental state, behaviour, and volition through interacting with André from his initial request (as well as using their previous knowledge of him to assist in their ongoing review of his level of risk). This would be examined in relation to concerns about potential relapse and also whether any changes in his speech or behaviour correspond to warning signs as documented in André's risk assessment (which would also be recorded in a truncated version in his care plan).

Reflective activity 8.9

Identify an example of aggressive behaviour from your clinical experience and describe the verbal (language used, volume, tone, pace of speech, threats) and non-verbal (appearance, eye contact, gestures, proximity to you or others, restlessness, acts of violence towards objects, other people or self) signs that demonstrated the person's expression of frustration, anger, and hostility. How would you know, from observing this person, when the risk of aggressive behaviour had subsided?

Standardized decision-making (cs2)

Service users are gradually given increased freedom. This follows a standardized procedure in forensic mental health care, giving staff (especially nursing staff) the opportunity to ascertain what effect these changes have had on André's physical, mental, social and behavioural states. This would be part of the risk management plan and is likely to include a summary of all identified risks that may take place as well as proposals for dealing with these potential risks should they arise (DH 2007b). Standardized risk assessment tools such as the HCR-20 (Webster et al. 1997) or GRiST (Buckingham 2007) might be used to assist in André's risk assessment and management plan. Although it is an ongoing debate, it is still considered preferable for nurses to focus their assessment of risk factors through observation and interaction rather than relying primarily on any actuarial risk tool (Silver and Miller 2002). It is also important that nurses are aware of the Mental Health Act 1983 governing André's in-patient care and treatment, and the restrictions imposed on André and the clinical team specified in various sections of this legislation (NICE 2005).

Reflective decision-making (cs2)

The fact that the request will be examined and formulated over a period of time allows all staff the opportunity to reflect upon the appropriateness of the request and the other options that could be available (Grounds 1995). It may be that André could be allowed a greater amount of unescorted leave within the hospital grounds. Usually, the care plan would guide the ongoing development of the treatment and any subsequent reflection would focus on André's behavioural and cognitive responses to each relaxation of the security surrounding his care, and the implications of this.

Reflective activity 8.10

When reviewing individual care plans how can you ensure that evaluations of patient progress and perceived outcomes of risk management strategies, accurately reflect what has actually occurred?

Ethical sensitivity in decision-making (cs2)

It is the responsibility of all staff to be sensitive, competent and aware of the different racial, faith, age, gender, disability and sexual information diversities that they come into contact with in their professional role (Chaloner 2000b). Therefore, any nursing contact should be value-free and André should be offered optimum care from all of the nurses on the ward. Nurses' responsibilities lie with their professional obligation to provide care and treatment for André. This means that they will not have any contact with the family and/or friends of the family whose flat André had set alight. This is different from the USA, where forensic nursing also encompasses victim support work (Burrow 1993). In the UK, the focus is on caring for the service user and their family (though if a family member was also a victim, there would be some involvement from the nursing team). This could be difficult for some members of the nursing team as those who are parents might find it difficult to distance themselves from feeling a great deal of sympathy for the victims. There is also a requirement to keep views, opinions and information about André confidential. The fact that the story aroused local interest may well mean that the media, local services and friends and family of the victims might all want information about André's care and treatment. A clear method for dealing with any requests for information would be agreed by the clinical team and unit management and it is imperative that nurses refer any requests via the agreed route, such as NHS trust press officer. It is also incumbent upon nurses to ensure that they do not reveal any confidential information to anyone within the local area. Although the information may be minor, there is always a potential of this information being leaked to a wider audience and it may lead to unforeseen consequences.

Accountability in decision-making (cs2)

Information regarding NMC accountability, recorded in John's case study, also applies to nurses' decision-making regarding André's care, as nurses use their professional knowledge, judgement and skills to make decisions based on evidence, good practice, and the person's best interests (NMC 2008). It is acknowledged that nurses will be involved in developing and evaluating a risk management strategy where the skills they use are centred on preventing any negative event from happening, and if this is not achievable, that the event results in the minimum amount of harm possible (DH 2007b). The nurses are accountable for ensuring that André receives the best care possible and that his safety, as well as the safety of everyone in the ward and wider community, is maintained. When making decisions about whether to support André's request, or not, nurses are required to ensure that their professional knowledge is sufficient to be able to make a valid independent evaluation. If their judgement is subsequently seen to be at fault or their level of knowledge is insufficient, they could be subject to both professional misconduct charges and potentially to legal redress. Although rare, if a serious untoward incident happens involving a person who is under the care of mental health services, a formal inquiry is now legally required. The inquiry has the power to summons anyone involved in the care of the service user and can make recommendations regarding legal proceedings that might be required if a professional is perceived to be at fault. Therefore, nurses will be formally accountable for their role in all risk assessment and risk management decisions from both a professional and legal perspective. A decision-making matrix indicating the pattern of nurses' responses to André is shown in Table 8.4.

Reflective activity 8.11

How can your clinical area reduce the risk of abuse and physical harm to patients, visitors and staff?

Table 8.4 Matrix of decisions made in relation to Case study 2

	PERCEPTIONS OF CLINICAL DECISION-MAKING									
CONCEPTIONS OF NURSING	Collaborative	Experience & Intuition	Confidence	Systematic	Prioritizing	Observation	Standardized	Reflective	Ethical Sensitivity	Accountability
Caring										
Listening & being there										
Practical procedures										
Knowledge & understanding										
Communicating										
Patience										
Teamwork										
Paperwork										
Empathizing & nonjudgemental										
Professional										

A matrix model of risk assessment/management in forensic mental health nursing

The actions and responses of the nursing staff in the two case studies are those that are expected of experienced nurses in secure settings. Tables 8.3 and 8.4 indicate that all of the clinical decision-making and conceptions of nursing characteristics are used by mental health nurses when assessing and managing the risk of aggressive or violent behaviour, both in short-term and long-term situations. Therefore, those nurses who are proficient in this area would appear to be utilizing all of the clinical decision-making skills noted by Standing (2007). The matrix model, as summarized in Tables 8.3 and 8.4, therefore offers a realistic representation of the wide range and different types of decision-making by forensic mental health nurses in these two clinical situations.

A comparison of the pattern of responses illustrated in Tables 8.3 and 8.4 indicates a difference between short- and long-term risk assessment/ management. A smaller range of decision-making characteristics is associated with what is perceived to be an imminent risk, as nurses use core skills necessary to deal with the current situation. Other decision-making skills are more likely to be used once the imminent risk has subsided. This view is supported by the fact that prioritizing was the only decision-making skill used more in Case study 1 than in Case study 2, as the decisions and interventions had to ensure the immediate safety and security of all those in the ward community. All the characteristics of clinical decision-making in the matrix model, except accountability and prioritizing, are used more in Case study 2 than in Case study 1. This may be due to having more time to examine options, consult, and reflect upon information regarding long-term risk assessment and management. In both case studies awareness of professional and/or legal accountability for decisions was evident and cross-referenced to each conception of nursing, indicating that this is a core aspect of both the short- and long-term risk assessment/management of aggressive behaviour.

Summary

This chapter has explored short- and long-term risk assessment and management of aggressive, abusive, threatening or potentially violent behaviour in the context of forensic mental health nursing. Different types of aggressive behaviour were related to corresponding levels of secure hospital environments to safely contain, treat and rehabilitate service users. The unique aspects of forensic mental health nursing were associated with caring for seriously mentally ill people who may also have a criminal history; mental health legislation governing compulsory treatment and security restrictions; locked in-patient secure ward/unit settings; and combining psychotherapeutic and custodial roles.

The expertise of this nursing specialty in preventing and managing violent behaviour can help to inform other areas of healthcare since aggressive behaviour can occur anywhere. Environmental, relational and procedural security was described as a guide to the prevention and management of aggressive behaviour in clinical practice. The matrix model was applied to analyse and compare clinical judgement and decision-making in short- and long-term risk assessment and management. It highlighted nurses' use of a wide range of decision-making skills, particularly for long-term risks, prioritizing was a key skill for immediate risks, and both short- and long-term risk assessment and management were strongly associated with professional and legal accountability for decisions and actions. Reflective activities were included throughout to encourage readers to understand and apply the principles and skills discussed to enhance safe healthcare in their own clinical practice.

Key points

- Aggression and/or violence can manifest in any healthcare environment so it is important to assess and manage risks, and forensic mental health care has expertise in this respect.
- Environmental security: Assess risks in the design and maintenance of buildings in providing a safe and secure setting to protect patients and staff, and enable observation and treatment.
- Relational security: Assess risks in the skill mix and staff–patient ratio, time available for face-to-face contact, and the quality of therapeutic rapport between staff and patients.
- Procedural security: Assess adequacy of policies, procedures and practices in controlling risks in relation to patients, members of staff, and the institution/hospital as a whole.
- Environmental/relational/procedural issues apply to other risk assessment e.g. infection control.
- Matrix model perceptions of decision-making/conceptions of nursing are representative of the knowledge and skills that were integrated and applied in short- and long-term risk assessment.

References

Bowers, L. (2002) *Dangerous and Severe Personality Disorder: Response and role of the psychiatric team.* London: Routledge.

Buckingham, C. (2007) Improving mental health risk assessment using web-based decision support. *Health Care Risk Report*, 13(3): 17–18.

Burrow, S. (1993) An outline of the forensic nursing role. *British Journal of Nursing*, 2, 899–904.

Chaloner, C. (2000a) Characteristics, skills knowledge and inquiry, in C. Chaloner and M. Coffey (eds) *Forensic Psychiatric Nursing: Current concepts.* Oxford: Blackwell Publishing, pp. 1–20.

Chaloner, C. (2000b) Ethics and morality, in C. Chaloner and M. Coffey (eds) *Forensic Psychiatric Nursing: Current concepts*. Oxford: Blackwell Publishing, pp. 269–87.

Department of Health (DH) (2007a) *Best Practice Guidance: Specification for adult medium-secure services*. London: DH.

Department of Health (DH) (2007b) *Best Practice in Managing Risk: Principles and evidence for best practice in the assessment and management of risk to self-and others in mental health services*. London: DH.

Faulk, M. (2000) *Basic Forensic Psychiatry*. Oxford: Blackwell Scientific Publications.

Grounds, A. (1995) Risk assessment and management in clinical context, in J. Crichton (ed.) *Psychiatric Patient Violence: Risk and response*. London: Duckworth, pp. 43–59.

Holloway, F. (1998) Risk assessment. *British Journal of Psychiatry*, 173(12): 540–3.

Kennedy, H. (2002) Therapeutic uses of security: mapping forensic mental health services by stratifying risk. *Advances in Psychiatric Treatment*, 8: 433–43.

MacInnes, D. (2000) *Risk Assessment in Mental Health*. Nursing Times Clinical Monograph No 47. London: Emap.

Mueser, K., Corrigan, P., Hilton, D. et al. (2004) Illness management and recovery: a review of the research. *Focus*, 4 (2): 34–47.

National Institute for Health and Clinical Excellence (NICE) (2005) *The Published Clinical Guideline on the Short-Term Management of Disturbed/Violent Behaviour in In-Patient Psychiatric Settings and Emergency Departments*. London: NICE.

Nolan, P., Dallender, J., Soares, J., Thomsen, S. and Arnetz, B. (1999) Violence in Mental Health Care: The experiences of mental health nurses and psychiatrists. *Journal of Advanced Nursing*, 30(4): 934–41.

Nursing and Midwifery Council (NMC) (2008) *The Code: Standards of conduct, performance and ethics for nurses and midwives*. London: NMC.

Pierzchniak, P., Farnham, F., De Taranto, N., et al. (1999) Assessing the needs of patients in secure settings: a multi-disciplinary approach. *Journal of Forensic Psychiatry*, 10(2): 343–54.

Quirk, A., Lelliott, P. and Seale, C. (2004) Service users' strategies for managing risk in the volatile environment of an acute psychiatric ward. *Social Science and Medicine*, 59(12): 2573–83.

Reed, J. (1992) *Final Summary Report. Review of Health and Social Services for Mentally Disordered Offenders and Others Requiring Similar Services*. London: HMSO.

Royal College of Psychiatrists (1998) *Management of Imminent Violence: Clinical practice guidelines for support mental health services*. Occasional Paper OP41. London: Royal College of Psychiatrists.

Scott, P. (1977) Assessing dangerousness in criminals. *British Journal of Psychiatry*, 131: 127–42.

Scottish Forensic Network (2007) *Definition of Security Levels in Psychiatric Inpatient Facilities in Scotland*. www.forensicnetwork.scot.nhs.uk/documents/previous_reports/levelsofsecurityreport.doc

Silver, E. and Miller, L. (2002) A cautionary note on the use of actuarial risk assessment tools for social control. *Crime and Delinquency*, 48: 138–61.

Standing, M. (2007) Clinical decision-making skills on the developmental journey from student to registered nurse: a longitudinal inquiry. *Journal of Advanced Nursing*, 60(3): 257–69.

Swinton, J. and Boyd, J. (1999) Autonomy and personhood: the forensic nurse as a moral agent, in D. Robinson and A. Kettles (eds) *Forensic Nursing and Multidisciplinary Care of the Mentally Disordered Offender*. London: Jessica Kingsley, pp. 128–41.

Tennant, A. et al. (2000) Working with the personality disordered offender, in C. Chaloner and M. Coffey (eds) *Forensic Psychiatric Nursing: Current Concepts*. Oxford: Blackwell Publishing, pp. 94–117.

UKCC (1999) *Nursing in Secure Environments*. London: UKCC.

Vinestock, M. (1996) Risk assessment. 'A word to the wise'. *Advances in Psychiatric Treatment*, 2: 3–10.

Webster, C., Douglas, K., Eaves, D. and Hart, S. (1997) *HCR-20. Assessing Risk for Violence. Version 2*. Burnaby, British Columbia: Mental Health Law and Policy Institute.

Whittington, R. and Wykes, T. (1996) An evaluation of staff training in psychological techniques for the management of patient violence. *Journal of Clinical Nursing*, 5(4): 257–61.

APPENDIX 8.1

Broad categories for high, medium and low security (Scottish Forensic Network 2007)

High Security – is the level of security necessary only for those service users who pose a grave and immediate danger to others if at large. Security arrangements should be capable of preventing even the most determined absconder. High secure services should only be provided in secure hospitals with a full range of therapeutic and recreational facilities within the perimeter fence, acknowledging the severe limitations on the use of outside services and facilities.

Medium Security – is the level of security necessary for service users who represent a serious but less immediate danger to others. Service users will often have been dealt with in the Crown Courts and present a serious risk to others combined with the potential to abscond. Security should therefore be sufficient to deter all but the most determined. A good range of therapeutic and recreational facilities should be available within the perimeter fence to meet the needs of service users who are not ready for off-site parole, but with the emphasis on graduated use of ordinary community facilities in rehabilitation whenever possible.

Low Security – is the level of security deemed necessary for service users who present a less serious physical danger to others, often dealt with in the Magistrates Courts and identified by court assessment/diversion schemes. Security measures are intended to impede rather than completely prevent absconding, with greater reliance on staffing arrangements and less reliance on physical security measures.

Reflecting on judgement and decisions in clinical supervision

Susan Plummer and Hesham Hassan

Overview

This chapter reflects on a clinical supervision session within primary mental health care in which the revised cognitive continuum – nine modes of practice (Chapter 5) is used as a guide to discuss judgement and decision-making. It explores the value of clinical supervision in nursing and interprofessional healthcare to reflect upon practice, analyse judgements, decisions and actions, and in enabling continuing professional development and application of these skills in everyday practice. The clinical supervision process and reflective learning cycle are used to structure an exploration of judgement and decision-making which is analysed with reference to the nine modes of practice. It is argued that cognitive continuum theory can increase supervisors' awareness of supervisees' needs, which in turn influences the development of the supervision process. Principles of supervision and reflective practice are relevant to all areas of healthcare, and reflective activities encourage readers to apply contents to enhance their own clinical practice.

Objectives

- Appreciate the value of clinical supervision in reflecting on clinical judgement/decision-making
- Identify managerial, educational and supportive functions of supervision to enhance practice
- Apply cognitive continuum theory in clinical supervision to analyse judgement/decisions/action
- Consider use of cognitive continuum theory to enhance supervisor-supervisee understanding
- Reflect and relate clinical supervision/cognitive continuum theory to own clinical practice area

Models of supervision

Systems of healthcare delivery and interprofessional practice are continuously changing (Chapter 3) and this leads to practitioners having more autonomy, independence and responsibility. In order to continually adjust to the demands of new working practices health professionals need to develop new skills and be accountable to patients, public, and their profession. One of the support mechanisms in place for this is clinical supervision (Chapter 4) but the number benefiting varies greatly between disciplines and areas of the country, according to Butterworth et al. (2008). Their review of clinical supervision literature from 2001 to 2007 reports that clinical supervision develops a deeper awareness of thinking and decision-making (Spence et al. 2002); increases problem solving ability (Zorga 2002); facilitates change in current practice (Cheater and Hale 2001; Willson et al. 2001); and enables nurses to become more ethically sensitive (Severinsson 2001). The impact on patient outcomes is less clear (Carson 2007) and more research is needed. In Wales, a survey of 815 mental health nurses, using the Manchester Clinical Supervision Scale (Winstanley 2000), found that clinical supervision was most positively evaluated when it was delivered monthly for at least 45 minutes and up to one hour duration (Edwards et al. 2005).

There are a variety of models of clinical supervision, individual supervision being the most common arrangement in nursing (Duarri and Kendrick 1999; Jones and Bennett 1998). No single model fulfils the needs of all clinical contexts (Fowler 1996) and so healthcare organizations may use elements of more than one model. Sloan and Watson (2002) claim Proctor's (1987) three-function interactive model (see Chapter 4) is the most frequently used supervision model in the United Kingdom, and its use is recommended in mental health nursing (Cottrell 2001; Faugier 1996). Other useful models include: six category intervention analysis (Heron 1989); problem-focused (Rogers and Topping-Morris 1997); solution-focused (Driscoll 2000); cognitive therapy derived (Beck 1976; Weishaar 1993; Padesky 1996); and practice-centred clinical supervision (Nicklin 1997).

Nicklin's model is similar to Proctor's but reframes formative, normative and restorative functions as managerial, educational and supportive. Managerial functions focus on workload and time, educational functions facilitate reflective learning, and supportive functions help the supervisee to cope emotionally. Nicklin describes stages in the supervision cycle as practice analysis, problem identification, objective setting, planning, implementation, and evaluation. Educational functions of Nicklin's model can be complemented by applying cognitive therapy principles since these aim to enable recipients to learn and test new ways of thinking and resolving life problems. Padesky (1996) recommends that supervision reflects the structure of cognitive therapy by using pre-planned questions to structure and focus each supervision session, for example:

- Is there a cognitive model to understand and treat the problem and is this being followed?

- Does the therapist have the knowledge and skills to implement interventions effectively?
- Is the therapy progressing as one would expect or not?
- What might be interfering and how can this be addressed?

Supervision has to be focused, structured, educational and collaborative (Sloan and Watson 2002), and incorporating cognitive therapy principles can help facilitate this, particularly in certain areas of mental health care. It may not be as applicable in other areas of interprofessional healthcare that could benefit from a more generic framework to support the achievement of Sloan and Watson's supervision criteria. For example, use of Johns' (2000) reflective cycle to: identify incident/put into context, reflect, identify alternative action, and discuss learning from the reflection. This chapter will also apply and review revised cognitive continuum theory (Chapter 5) within clinical supervision.

Reflective activity 9.1

If you currently receive clinical supervision:

- Reflect on its strengths and weaknesses in helping you to develop clinical practice and write this down for future reference, for example, in relation to your personal/professional portfolio.
- Identify examples from your experience as a supervisee of each of the managerial, educational and supportive functions of clinical supervision regarding its effectiveness in enabling you to manage time and workload, learn new skills, and feel supported in your clinical practice.
- What do you need to do to benefit more from your future experience of clinical supervision?

If you do not currently receive clinical supervision:

- Imagine that a system of clinical supervision is being introduced in your area next week and make a list of all the reasons why it might be a good idea and why it might be a bad idea.
- Write down all the characteristics you would expect in an effective clinical supervisor and the rules that you think would be important for the supervisor-supervisee relationship to abide by.
- Reflect on managerial, educational and supportive functions of clinical supervision and identify issues where you need support in managing workload, learning skills, and sharing concerns.
- Discuss with colleagues and clinical manager the benefits of introducing clinical supervision.

Primary mental health care context

The clinical focus for supervision is a recently established multidisciplinary, preventative mental health care service provided by a primary care NHS trust.

It offers assessment, advice, and 'talking therapies' to treat anxiety, phobia, depression or behavioural problems as alternatives to or to complement tranquillizers and antidepressants general practitioners (GPs) might prescribe. GPs from various practices in the area make referrals to the service, which are allocated according to the nature of problems and expertise required at regular team meetings. The primary mental health care team consists of team leader, counsellors, psychologist, mental health worker, and mental health nurse, and each team member liaises with GPs regarding patient care. Patients who choose to use the service are usually seen within three weeks at a clinic in a local primary care centre. There is no medical specialist in the primary care team as it does not cater for patients with serious or long-term mental illness. These patients are seen by a community mental health team, provided by the local mental health NHS trust, including psychiatrists and a range of additional services.

Professional profile

The supervisee (Susan) was (at the time) a mental health nurse practitioner in the above primary mental health care team. My role was to carry out assessments, deliver brief interventions as necessary, liaise and advise GPs on appropriate treatment, and refer to other services as required. The supervisor (Hesham) is a consultant psychiatrist in a community mental health team from a neighbouring area who agreed to provide clinical supervision for an hour on a monthly basis. This interprofessional arrangement enabled me to benefit from Hesham's expertise in psychiatry and community mental health when reflecting on and developing my practice via clinical supervision.

The clinical supervision session

The clinical supervision session took place one week after a patient consultation described in the following case study. The case study is presented in relation to stages of the supervision cycle including practice analysis, problem identification, objective setting, planning, implementation, and evaluation (Nicklin 1997). The revised cognitive continuum – nine modes of practice (intuitive/reflective/patient and peer-aided/system-aided judgement – critical review of experiential/research evidence – clinical audit, action/qualitative/survey/experimental research) (Standing 2008) is used to analyse clinical judgement/decision-making and the actions taken. Finally, a reflective cycle (Johns 2000) of applying cognitive continuum theory within clinical supervision is discussed.

Case study

Emily (pseudonym) is a 19-year-old woman referred to the primary care mental health service by her GP. The referral letter stated she currently had a low mood and also a history of lacerating her arms and misusing laxatives. Previously, she had expressed thoughts of taking an overdose but the GP did not think she would act on these thoughts. Emily was prescribed antidepressant medication (selective serotonin reuptake inhibitor (SSRI) last year but without any apparent benefit.

Emily appeared well dressed with good personal hygiene but was tearful upon her arrival. She gave a history of her recent depression which she attributed to problems within her family. She currently felt very unsafe and said it was highly likely that she would attempt suicide that evening as she was going to be at home on her own for the weekend. She was tearful throughout the consultation. She said she recently split up with her boyfriend and had just been told by him that he refused to go back into a relationship with her. She told me that if he agreed to come back to her, she would not have thoughts of suicide and would probably not attempt to harm herself. Problems and risks identified included worsening symptoms of depression, alcohol misuse, binge eating and vomiting, family problems, history of deliberate self-harm, recent split from partner, current suicidal thoughts and intentions, and no immediate support apparently available from family or friends.

Objectives were discussed with Emily and prioritized according to the perceived risks. Given her expressed suicidal intentions, history of vulnerability, and recent traumatic events, Emily's safety was the immediate priority which she herself acknowledged. Once this had been achieved, longer-term objectives for Emily would be to explore treatment options for the underlying depression she appeared to experience, reduce her alcohol consumption, address her binge eating and vomiting, curtail further acts of deliberate self-harm and explore contributing factors such as her relationship with her family members, relationships with partners, and sense of guilt over her parents' divorce.

Emily agreed she did not feel safe enough to be on her own that night or the coming weekend but refused to call her mother to tell of her distress. She insisted she would be safe if her ex-partner returned but acknowledged he felt that she was emotionally blackmailing him. I discussed with Emily the advisability of referring her to: the community mental health service including crisis team to monitor her safety in the short term; self-harm team to help her address her pattern of self-harming behaviour; and to a practice counsellor to explore other ways of dealing with her troubles. I also planned to talk to the GP about reviewing antidepressant medication and doing blood tests to check any physiological causes and/or effects of her vomiting, poor nutrition and depression.

When I spoke to the community mental health team on the phone they were unable to carry out an urgent home assessment on that day but could see Emily at their centre. I decided the safest option was to escort Emily to their centre where she was assessed and able to return to her home that day with support from the crisis team. I later talked to the GP who prescribed a new course of antidepressants which in due course appeared to benefit Emily. She attended the self-harm service and practice counsellor, and, six months following the initial assessment, Emily's GP informed me she had stopped harming herself, stopped binge eating and vomiting, and her alcohol consumption had also reduced. She continued to see the practice counsellor for support and to explore new ways of coping with stress and her relationship problems.

Applying revised cognitive continuum – nine modes of practice to review decisions

Task structure and cognitive modes

Cognitive continuum theory combines a continuum of decision tasks varying in complexity from low to high structure, with a continuum of cognitive modes ranging from intuition to analysis. The nine modes of practice described by Standing (2008) are the product of interaction between the two systems that link theory to practice in clinical decision-making (Chapter 5, Figure 5.3). As Hamm (1988) points out, the nature of the decision task a clinician is working on is important in determining the kind of thinking and most appropriate cognitive mode that needs to be adopted and, in turn, the type of decision made. Standing (2008) associates less structured tasks with subjective 'face-to-face' decisions and more structured tasks with objective 'faceless' decisions, arguing that the former prompts intuition and the latter prompts analysis in thinking and cognition. More effective decision-making is thought to result from effectively matching the most relevant cognitive mode to the particular demands and complexity of each decision task. The structure of decision tasks during Emily's consultation and assessment therefore needs to be explored.

A range of decision tasks in Emily's consultation included assessing, planning and delivering care. We thought that these tasks ranged from low to midway on the continuum as they involve face-to-face decisions, suggesting that cognition was closer to intuition than analysis. Hammond (1996) associates intuition with forming ideas, opinions and decisions rapidly, without an awareness of the underlying process informing them. This does not preclude the possibility that the person has an extensive knowledge base, albeit mainly tacit knowledge and understanding from prior experience (Hamm 1988). The more time allowed by the nature of decision tasks the more opportunities there are for conscious deliberation, reflection, consideration of explicit knowledge, and increasing levels of analysis open to scrutiny and checking by others. Decision tasks requiring greater analysis are, therefore, more time-consuming than those requiring intuition. For example, patient assessments are allocated one hour but in Emily's case, due to her acute mental state and suicide risk, planning care became more highly structured requiring more analysis and it took more time. Consequently, in prioritizing urgent arrangements for Emily's continuing care, I exceeded the allocated time for her consultation which meant I had to negotiate rescheduling the following patient's appointment.

The changing nature of decision tasks therefore requires flexibility in clinical decision-making to respond appropriately. Hammond (1981) argues this is possible where cognition is not polarized at either end of an intuition-analysis continuum but continually oscillating back and forth in varying combinations, as represented in healthcare by the nine modes of practice (Standing 2008).

Nine modes of practice

In discussing Emily's case study during clinical supervision we looked at each of the nine modes of practice and used them to interpret and analyse my clinical judgement/decision-making and action. Decision tasks prompting intuitive judgement include managing unexpected situations for which routine procedures appear inadequate to manage, and so stretch practitioners' coping skills (Hammond 1981; Hamm 1988; Standing 2008). In Emily's case, the letter from the GP stated she had experienced suicidal thoughts in the past but there was no indication that she was at risk now, so the acute level of her apparent distress and the expression of current suicidal intent were unexpected. As I had not met her before, and had no access to her GP or to her practice records at the clinic where I saw her, I only had Emily's self-report and my initial impressions of her to work with. My intuitive judgement was that Emily was likely to attempt suicide regardless of whether it would be a serious attempt or a 'cry for help' designed to persuade her boyfriend to come back to her.

I was then encouraged to think about how reflection-in-action (Schön 1987) had occurred during my consultation with Emily. I remembered being conscious of piecing together the risk factors of Emily's history of self-harm and suicidal thoughts, family problems, break-up with her boyfriend, social isolation, current level of distress and expression of suicidal intent. The culmination of these factors supported my intuitive feeling that she was at risk of attempting suicide. In reflecting-on-action (Schön 1987) during supervision my immediate priority had been to ensure Emily received adequate observation and support as I did not consider it was safe to ignore her acute distress and suicidal thoughts. In the longer term I considered she needed to be helped to learn new ways of thinking, behaving and relating to others especially when experiencing disappointments, stress, and depressive thoughts.

Patient and peer-aided judgement involves respecting patients' preference and right to participate in decision-making. It was important I collaborated with Emily as she was the main informant to guide my decision-making, and because she needed to be agreeable to the plan of care. I judged that Emily's depressive and suicidal thoughts were a serious risk that warranted more intensive observation and treatment than primary mental health care was equipped to provide, and this is why I sought peer-aided judgement and assistance from the community mental health service. Once they had assessed Emily, she was followed up by the crisis and self-harm teams, suggesting her referral to the community mental health service was justified. I also collaborated with the GP in reviewing Emily's antidepressant medication and in referring her to the practice counsellor.

System-aided judgement involves applying validated clinical assessment tools and guidelines, and represents a shift along the cognitive continuum towards more explicit forms of knowledge and analytical thinking. I was aware of tools such as the Patient Health Questionnaire (Kroenke et al. 2001) and Beck Depression Inventory (Beck et al. 1988) which could be used to structure Emily's mental health assessment. I did not apply them directly as Emily was too distressed; they require mental concentration and sufficient time to complete properly, and it was already evident that Emily was experiencing a moderate to severe level of depression. Indirectly, such tools did help to inform and support my identification and understanding of risk factors highlighted in Emily's assessment.

Critical review of experiential and research evidence is positioned midway on the revised cognitive continuum between the four judgement-based and four research-based practice modes (Chapter 5, Figure 5.3). In reviewing experiential evidence of applying judgement-based practice modes (intuitive, reflective, patient and peer-aided, system-aided) I became more aware of the differences between them and the progression in analytical thinking when moving from intuitive to system-aided judgement. In reviewing my decision-making, I cannot be certain that Emily would have attempted or committed suicide if I had not instituted the short- and longer-term care arrangements. On reflection the measures taken appear appropriate in relation to the problems presented by Emily, and her reported progress seems to support this. Given the range of short-term/longer-term interventions applied it is difficult to attribute progress to any single therapy, and it is probable that Emily benefited from their combined effect. How lasting this may be is difficult to predict and a test of how well Emily has learnt to cope will arise when her counselling sessions come to an end.

In reviewing evidence of applying research-based practice modes (clinical audit/action, qualitative, survey, experimental), I did not apply any of them directly since I was focused on my practitioner role in helping Emily, not researching her care. But, indirectly, they were applied in the 'critical review of experiential and research evidence' practice mode through an awareness and application of relevant research-based literature. For example, the assessment tools referred to earlier in system-aided judgement are derived from survey research. This helped me to recognize risk factors regarding Emily's safety, including evidence of depression, traumatic life events, social isolation, history of self-harm, suicidal thoughts/intentions (and that previous attempts significantly increase the risk of suicide). I was also aware that national guidelines (NICE 2004a) recommend SSRI antidepressant medication (which was developed via experimental research and controlled trials), the same type Emily had previously been prescribed, for patients with moderate to severe depression and/or symptoms of bulimia nervosa, such as binge eating and self-induced vomiting (NICE 2004b). Emily said she stopped taking them after two weeks as she did not feel they had any effect on her mood. I was able to inform her that it takes three to four weeks for the tablets to start working so she should try taking them for longer to feel the benefits.

NICE (2004 a, b) also recommend combining SSRI antidepressants with cognitive behaviour therapy (CBT) for patients who are depressed and/or bulimic, which fitted Emily's profile. However, I was not sufficiently skilled in this particular therapy and there was no locally based CBT practitioner available, despite the wide range of interprofessional mental health workers employed. In other words, a relevant cognitive model was available to treat Emily's condition but there was a lack of an appropriately trained therapist (Padesky 1996). It suggests that the skill mix needs reviewing, for example, training and supervision could help to develop local CBT practitioners. Reviewing the adequacy of available mental health care services reflects elements of the clinical audit/action research practice mode. As the treatment of choice was unavailable, I organized alternative counselling sessions to provide a psychological complement to Emily's new biochemical regime of antidepressants prescribed by the GP. This was in addition to the involvement of the community mental health service for immediate/short-term monitoring of her mental state/safety and modifying her self-harm behaviour. A network of agencies was therefore coordinated for Emily, contributing to effective whole systems working and collaboration between practitioners in different subsystems to provide integrated, responsive, patient-centred 'joined up care' (Chapter 3).

Reflective activity 9.2

Work through the following with your clinical supervisor. If you do not have a clinical supervisor, choose a suitable colleague you would like to work with on this activity.

1. Think about your own role as a healthcare practitioner, identify a range of decision tasks you deal with, discuss their complexity, and list them from lower to higher structured tasks.
2. Compare/contrast lower-higher structured tasks in relation to your application of experiential or research-based knowledge, intuitive or analytical thinking, and time needed to make decisions.
3. Apply the nine modes of practice to analyse your clinical judgement/decision-making regarding a patient you have cared for, discuss any managerial, educational and support issues arising from this in relation to organization/delivery of care, and your professional development needs.
4. Discuss and write down an action plan to address the issues identified above specifying aims, objectives, action to be taken, date to review progress, and criteria to check achievements.

Reflecting on applying the revised cognitive continuum within clinical supervision

We discussed our experience of applying the revised cognitive continuum – nine modes of practice during clinical supervision to analyse my clinical judgement/decision-making in Emily's care. Standing (2008) claims 'the revised cognitive continuum encompasses patient-centred judgement tasks, collaborative, ethical, reflective, qualitative and quantitative evidence-based practice and professional accountability' (p. 20). We felt that by using the continuum, we were able to discuss these issues in relation to judgements, decisions and interventions used in clinical practice. As healthcare professionals are increasingly expected to review, develop and apply judgement/decision-making skills, we concluded the revised cognitive continuum is a valuable tool to examine the relationship between decision tasks, ways of thinking about them, and action strategies. Other devices, such as the reflective learning cycle (Johns 2000) are also useful but do not provide as detailed, in-depth, or breadth of analysis and evaluation, in relation to the decision-making process.

Hammond (1980) argued that a person's reasoning is more effective when adopting the mode of thinking that corresponds to the task features and if a decision task requires analytical cognition but the clinician deals with it intuitively, errors can occur. For example, Emily intuitively felt that the antidepressants were not working after a couple of weeks of taking them and so she decided to stop. By sharing with her an informed analysis of the time required to develop therapeutic levels of the medication in her system she understood the reason why she had not felt any benefit before, and that she needed to take the tablets for a longer period for them to be effective. Errors can also occur if a decision task requires intuition but the clinician deals with it analytically. For example, if I had asked Emily to complete a highly structured assessment tool to analyse her depression, it would have been difficult to complete in her emotional state, and I would have been distracted from attending to vital information cues in her verbal/non-verbal behaviour. In this way our reflection on applying the revised cognitive continuum illustrated to us how clinical supervision can promote awareness of the need to match decision tasks to the most appropriate practice mode.

Social and organizational contexts also influence clinicians' judgement and decision-making via different expectations and educational experiences (Hamm et al. 1984) and require consideration during clinical supervision. For example, Hamm (1988) discusses medical reasoning in hospital ward rounds involving those with different levels of experience and education. We inferred that this also meant they would be at different stages in terms of their analytical ability and their knowledge base within each of the nine modes of practice. For the purpose of clinical supervision, this reinforced to us the need for supervisor and supervisee to be aware of their differences in expertise and for the supervisor to adopt a mode on the intuition/analysis continuum that was matched with the supervisee's learning needs. This means that the supervisor needs to be familiar with the supervisee's educational and professional background as a basis for helping to extend the supervisee's range of intuitive and analytical skills. We felt that both supervisors and supervisees would benefit from professional development and training in applying the revised cognitive continuum to enhance effective judgement/decision-making within clinical supervision.

We found that the revised cognitive continuum can also be used to analyse the clinical supervision process itself. We felt that clinical supervision as a task structure is probably in the middle of the 'low' to 'high' range and corresponds with the critical review of experiential/research evidence practice mode. This enables a review of all the judgement-based and research-based practice modes used in relation to the various decision tasks discussed. Applying the revised cognitive continuum enabled us to consider not only the supervisee's thinking and decision-making, but also the thinking and reasoning that occurred during the clinical supervision session. This, in itself, was an educational opportunity which enhanced analytical thinking and a deeper understanding of the relationship between cognition and action, and its application in day-to-day clinical practice.

Although this chapter has reflected on a case study in a mental health context, the process of clinical supervision is relevant and applicable to practitioners in any healthcare context. Nurses and other healthcare professionals are required to develop and apply effective clinical judgement and decision-making skills in their interventions with patients/clients/service users. Clinical supervision supports ongoing professional development of such skills, and incorporating the revised cognitive continuum within clinical supervision complements practitioners' lifelong learning in this respect.

Summary

This chapter has discussed the value of clinical supervision in continuing professional development and lifelong learning of practitioners' clinical decision-making skills. Models of supervision were outlined and managerial, educational and supportive functions were identified that can enhance practitioners' clinical practice. An example was described of an actual supervision session that discussed and reviewed a case study of the practitioners' recent consultation with a vulnerable patient. The revised cognitive continuum – nine modes of practice was applied during clinical supervision to analyse clinical judgement/decision-making and subsequent interventions.

The revised cognitive continuum can be used to guide both the process of clinical supervision and as a tool to examine the thinking, judgement and decisions made during patient care. The task structure within the consultation needs to be identified and matched with the nine modes of practice which are distributed along a cognitive continuum ranging from intuition to analysis. The case study was examined regarding the transparency of decision process, the time required to complete decision tasks, and the selection of suitable modes of practice. The revised cognitive continuum stimulates both intuitive and analytic thinking within the process of supervision and it was found that applying the continuum positively affects the supervision process. Usually clinical supervision involves working through an analysis of clinical practice, then identifying points for exploration, examining decisions that are made, identifying alternative actions, and reflecting on the outcomes and learning. Applying the revised cognitive continuum complemented this process and enabled a deeper level of reflection and development of clinical judgement and decision-making skills. While the revised cognitive was applied in the context of primary mental health care, it could be combined and applied via clinical supervision for practitioners in any healthcare setting. Reflective activities were included to help readers apply the principles to their own clinical practice. We concluded that the revised cognitive continuum is a useful tool to guide clinical supervision and its inclusion could enhance supervisor training programmes. Further evaluation of its application is recommended in terms of impact on supervisee development and on patient care outcomes. This could contribute to existing evidence in the use of clinical supervision to enhance clinical practice.

Key points

- Clinical supervision has three main functions: restorative – offer emotional support; formative – facilitate reflective learning; and normative – monitor work load and quality issues.
- Benefits of clinical supervision include: develop critical thinking and decision-making; increase problem solving ability; facilitate changes in practice; and develop ethical awareness/sensitivity.
- A clinical supervision cycle involves: practice analysis, problem identification, objective setting, planning, implementation, and evaluation, e.g. review practitioner's care of a suicidal patient.
- Clinical supervision is more effective when focused, structured, educational and collaborative.
- Applying cognitive continuum theory – nine modes of practice in clinical supervision enables a review of practitioners' decision tactics which may identify areas for professional development.

References

Beck, A.T. (1976) *Cognitive Therapy and the Emotional Disorders*. New York: New York International University Press.

Beck, A.T., Steer, R.A. and Garbin, M.G. (1988) Psychometric properties of the Beck Depression Inventory: twenty-five years of evaluation. *Clinical Psychology Reviews*, 8: 77–100.

Butterworth, T., Bell, L., Jackson, C. and Panjnkihar, M. (2008) Wicked spell or magic bullet? A review of the clinical supervision literature 2001–2007. *Nurse Education Today*, 28: 264–72.

Carson, J. (2007) Instruments for evaluating clinical supervision, in V. Bishop (ed.) *Clinical Supervision in Practice*, 2nd edn. Basingstoke: Palgrave Macmillan.

Cheater, F.M. and Hale, C. (2001) An evaluation of a local clinical supervision scheme for practice nurses. *Journal of Clinical Nursing*, 10: 119–31.

Cottrell, S. (2001) Occupational stress and job satisfaction in mental health nursing: focused interventions through evidence-based assessment. *Journal of Psychiatric and Mental Health Nursing*, 8: 157–64.

Driscoll, J. (2000) Clinical supervision: A radical approach. *Mental Health Practice, 3*: 8–10.

Duarri, W. and Kendrick, K. (1999) Implementing clinical supervision. *Professional Nurse*, 14: 849–52.

Edwards, D., Cooper, L., Burnard, P., et al. (2005) Factors influencing the effectiveness of clinical supervision. *Journal of Psychiatric and Mental Health Nursing*, 12: 405–41.

Faugier, J. (1996) Clinical supervision and mental health nursing, in T. Sandford and K. Gournay (eds) *Perspectives in Mental Health Nursing*. London: Bailliere Tindall.

Fowler, J. (1996) Clinical supervision: what do you do after you say hello? *British Journal of Nursing*, 5: 382–5.

Hamm, R.M. (1988) Clinical intuition and clinical analysis: expertise and the cognitive continuum, in J. Dowie and A. Elstein (eds) *Professional Judgement. A reader in clinical decision making*. Cambridge: Cambridge University Press.

Hamm, R.M., Clark, J.A. and Bursztajin, H. (1984) Psychiatrists' thorny judgments: describing and improving decision making processes. *Medical Decision Making*, 4: 425–47.

Hammond, K.R. (1980) *The Integration of Research in Judgment and Decision Theory* (Report 226) Boulder, CO: University of Colorado, Center for Research on Judgment and Policy.

Hammond, K.R. (1981) *Principles of Organisation in Intuitive and Analytical Cognition* (Report 231) Boulder, CO: University of Colorado, Center for Research on Judgment and Policy.

Hammond, K.R. (1996) *Human Judgement and Social Policy: Irreducible uncertainty, inevitable error, unavoidable injustice.* New York: Oxford University Press.

Heron, J. (1989) *Six Category Intervention Analysis.* Guildford: Human Potential Resource Group, University of Surrey.

Johns, C. (2000) *Becoming a Reflective Practitioner: A reflective and holistic approach to clinical nursing, practice development and clinical supervision.* Oxford: Blackwell Science.

Jones, A. and Bennett, J. (1998) Clinical supervision: A framework for practice. *Mental Health Practice*, 2: 18–22.

Kroenke, K., Spitzer, R.L. and Williams, J.B. (2001) The PHQ-9: validity of a brief depression severity measure. *Journal of General Intern Medicine*, 16: 606–13.

National Institute for Clinical Effectiveness (NICE) (2004a) *Depression: Management of depression in primary and secondary care – NICE guideline.* www.nice.org.uk/Guidance/CG23.

National Institute for Clinical Effectiveness (NICE) (2004b) *Eating Disorders: Core interventions in the treatment and management of anorexia, nervosa, bulimia nervosa and related eating disorders.* www.nice.org.uk/Guidance/CG9.

Nicklin, P. (1997) A practice-centred model of clinical supervision. *Nursing Times, 93*: 52–4.

Padesky, C. (1996) Developing cognitive therapist competency: Teaching and supervision models, in P. Salkovskis (ed.) *Frontiers of Cognitive Therapy*. London: Guilford Press.

Proctor, B. (1987) Supervision: A co-operative exercise in accountability, in M.M. and P.M. Leicester (eds) *Enabling and Ensuring: Supervision in practice.* National Youth Bureau and the Council for Education and Training in Youth and Community Work.

Rogers, P. and Topping-Morris, B. (1997) Clinical supervision for forensic mental health nurses. *Nursing Management,* 4: 13–15.

Schön, D.A. (1987) *Educating the Reflective Practitioner: Toward a new design of teaching and learning in the professions.* San Francisco: Jossey-Bass.

Severinsson, E.I. (2001) Confirmation, meaning and self-awareness as core concepts of the nursing supervision model. *Nursing Ethics,* 8: 36–44.

Sloan, G. and Watson, H. (2002) Clinical supervision models for nursing: Structure, research and limitations. *Nursing Standard,* 17: 41–6.

Spence, C., Cantrell, J., Christie, I. and Samet, W. (2002) A collaborative approach to the implementation of clinical supervision. *Journal of Nursing Management,* 10: 65–74.

Standing, M. (2008) Clinical judgement and decision-making in nursing – nine modes of practice in a revised cognitive continuum. *Journal of Advanced Nursing,* 62(1): 124–34.

Weishaar, M.E. (1993) *Aaron T. Beck.* London: Sage.

Willson, L., Fawcett, T. and Whyte, D.A. (2001) An evaluation of a clinical supervision programme. *British Journal of Community Nursing,* 6: 614–23.

Winstanley, J. (2000) Clinical supervision: Development of an evaluation instrument. Unpublished PhD thesis. Faculty of Medicine, Dentistry and Nursing, University of Manchester.

Zorga, S. (2002) Supervision: the process of lifelong learning in social and educational professions. *Journal of Interprofessional Care,* 16: 265–76.

10 Reflexive-pragmatism: logic, practicality, rigour and relevance

Mooi Standing and Michael Standing

Overview

This chapter provides a patient's view of clinical judgement/decision-making in relation to two episodes of acute medical care for the same illness over a ten-year period. Examples of good practice demonstrate effective application of coherence (logical) and correspondence (practical) competence, plus scientific and ecological validity (rigour and relevance) in diagnostic and treatment decisions. Examples of decision-making errors are associated with problems in applying the above skills and processes. In reflecting on ways to promote and perpetuate good practice in clinical judgement/decision-making, a new reflexive-pragmatism model is created. This relates the above concepts from cognitive continuum theory to both patient-centred care and practice-centred lifelong learning in interprofessional healthcare. It is argued that such a model can help to reduce a theory-practice gap, offer a coherent and practical philosophy of interprofessional healthcare, and can be applied by practitioners in reviewing and addressing their professional development needs.

Objectives

- Appreciate the experience of care delivery from an acutely ill patient's perspective
- Evaluate correspondence (practical) and coherence (logical) decision-making competence
- Apply scientific and ecological validity to assess rigour and relevance of clinical decisions
- Show how practical/logical skills plus checks of rigour/relevance relate to high quality care
- Apply reflexive-pragmatism to integrate patient-centred care and practice-centred learning
- Reflect on professional development needs in enhancing judgement/decision-making skills

Introduction

Like Chapters 6–9, this chapter uses real case studies to apply and discuss decision theory and research presented in Chapters 1–5. Unlike the case studies in Chapters 6–9, which were written from a practitioner's perspective, here they are based on first-hand experience as an acutely ill patient suffering from pulmonary embolism (blood clot in lung) in 1997 and 2007. The timeframe coincides with National Health Service (NHS) reform advocating high quality patient-centred care via clinical governance and evidence-based practice (Chapters 1–3), and, education reform that values practice-centred learning (Chapters 1 and 4). Comparing and contrasting the quality of care received provides one patient's perception of change that had taken place in diagnostic, treatment and nursing decisions. Practitioners' coherence (logical) and correspondence (practical) competence in clinical decision-making (Chapter 5), are evaluated and, surprisingly, the perceived quality of care was better in 1997 than in 2007. This suggests a theory–practice gap between the ideal (what practitioners say they should do) and the real (what they actually do), which is exacerbated by a philosophical and geographical separation of education from the management and delivery of healthcare (Maben et al. 2006).

As a nurse tutor, the experience of being a patient profoundly affected my perception of clinical judgement and decision-making, prompting me to reflect on ways to enhance the development and application of these skills by nurses and other health professionals. This resulted in my researching nurses' perceptions of clinical decision-making skills and in revising cognitive continuum theory for application in nursing and interprofessional healthcare (Chapters 1 and 5). What this chapter adds is a new reflexive-pragmatism model of patient-centred interprofessional healthcare that also emphasizes lifelong practice-centred learning in clinical judgement and decision-making. Reflexive-pragmatism involves developing and applying both coherence and correspondence competence to explain, justify and defend the logic of decision-making in relation to relevant theory, research and professional values, and to ensure decisions have the best possible clinical outcome for patients.

Reflexive-pragmatism reflects the strengths identified in the two case studies and indicates how potential weaknesses can be addressed in future practice. It combines elements of theory and research (Chapters 1 to 5) within a unified model of complementary opposites that includes scientific versus experiential processes, formal versus informal learning, and evidence-based versus reflective practice. It is hoped that this can help to reduce a theory–practice gap by offering educators, managers and practitioners a shared philosophy of lifelong learning in patient-centred, interprofessional healthcare. A summary/checklist is included, enabling practitioners to self-assess correspondence and coherence competence for continuing professional development purposes.

Case studies 1 and 2

Two episodes of the same potentially life-threatening illness (pulmonary embolism), occurring in the same person (Mooi), following long-haul air travel over a ten-year period are compared, contrasted, and summarized in Table 10.1. On both occasions the acute medical care (in the same hospital) resulted in the illness being successfully treated. The main differences between the two case studies lie in the accuracy of the general practitioner's (GP) provisional diagnosis, the perceived quality of nursing care received, and the presence or absence of additional medical complications.

Table 10.1 Comparison of Case study 1 and Case study 2

Points to compare	'Mooi' Case study 1 (1997)	'Mooi' Case study 2 (2007)
Precipitating factors	Air travel – long-haul return flight	Air travel – long-haul return flight
Symptoms	Chest pain, breathless, cough, hot sensation around back, tiredness	Chest pain, breathless, cough, hot sensation around back, tiredness
Self-provisional diagnosis	Chest infection	Pulmonary embolism
GP provisional diagnosis	Pulmonary embolism	Chest infection
GP treatment plan	Ambulance transfer to hospital	Review after 48 hours if no better
Hospital admission	Assessed straightaway in A&E and later transferred/treated in medical ward	Taken to hospital next day from work with severe chest pain, breathless and very pale; assessed/treated in A&E, clinical decision unit, and medical ward
Diagnostic tests	Arterial blood oxygen saturation and full computed tomography (CT) scan	Arterial blood oxygen saturation level and full CT scan to detect blood clots
Diagnosis	Pulmonary embolism	Pulmonary embolism
Initial treatment	Intravenous infusion, anticoagulant and fluids, painkillers, oxygen, rest	Intravenous/subcutaneous anticoagulant, painkillers, oxygen, rest
Perception of nursing care	Caring, task orientated	Uncaring, task orientated
Complications	None	Acute chest infection
Aftercare	Anticoagulant tablets for 6 months, blood monitored at out-patients clinic	3 consecutive courses of different antibiotics, anticoagulant tablets for 6 months, blood monitored at out-patients clinic, prophylactic anti-coagulant injections before and after all future long-haul flights

Analysis of clinical decision-making in Case studies 1 and 2

In both case studies I initially attended the same GP practice with similar symptoms. In 1997 I saw an experienced GP and in 2007 I saw an inexperienced GP. Despite having no previous history of pulmonary embolism in 1997 (when its risk on long-haul flights was not acknowledged by airlines) the GP correctly identified it as the provisional diagnosis (Table 10.2). Conversely, in 2007 (when airlines acknowledged it as a risk on long-haul flights and gave prevention advice), despite having a previous history of pulmonary embolism, and my saying the symptoms felt the same as last time, the GP incorrectly identified a chest infection as the provisional diagnosis. In order to understand how GP(1) obtained a more accurate provisional diagnosis than GP(2), correspondence (practical) and coherence (logical) competence (Hammond 1996; Standing 2008) are assessed, (previously discussed in Chapter 5) to analyse the two GPs' respective clinical decision-making skills.

Table 10.2 GP(1) correspondence and coherence competence – Case study 1

Correspondence competence	Coherence competence
Piecing together clues of presenting complaint	Systematic conduct of physical examination
Listening to patient's account of feeling unwell following long-haul flight; and how chest pain is related to other factors such as exertion, cough, breathlessness, and feeling hot on the back	Consideration of alternative potential conditions in relation to symptoms such as chest infection, pleurisy (inflamed lining of lung), pneumothorax (collapsed lung), or a problem with the heart
Using stethoscope to assess lungs/breathing	Understanding lung function, relating this to chest sounds, and excluding above conditions
Using electrocardiogram (ECG) to assess heart	Understanding heart function, relating this to the ECG result, and excluding a heart problem
Using pulse oximeter fingertip probe on index finger to assess oxygen (O2) saturation level	Understanding normal O2 saturation (>95%) and implications of below normal oximeter result
Observation of patient's demeanour, pallor, degree of discomfort and shortness of breath; and noting how this was made worse with a little exertion e.g. getting onto the examination couch	Understanding significance of signs, symptoms, and precipitating factors realize there is a high risk the symptoms are due to a pulmonary embolism and that it is a potentially life-threatening illness
Arrange urgent ambulance transfer to hospital	Explain reason for referral in letter to duty doctor

Reflective activity 10.1

Refer to the examples of correspondence (practical) competence and coherence (logical) competence in Table 10.2 and create two new tables with the same headings:

1. Reflect on your observation of good practice by a colleague when assessing a patient and describe examples of correspondence and coherence competence.

2. Reflect on an example from your own practice when assessing a patient and describe examples of correspondence and coherence competence you applied.

Table 10.2 illustrates the differences between correspondence and coherence competence and their interdependent contribution to effective clinical decision-making by GP(1). Correspondence competence applied practical or interpersonal skills to observe, elicit information, and assess patient health status to inform diagnostic and treatment decisions which were relevant to patient needs, and to optimize effective care outcomes. Coherence competence applied logical and theoretical skills to guide systematic problem solving, understand implications of observations regarding theory and research in health and illness, assess risks, and prioritize clinical decisions. Each contrasting but complementary skill set was effectively used and combined by GP(1) linking experiential/intuitive and analytic/rational decision-making (Chapter 5, Table 5.1), as cognitive continuum theory suggests, to fulfil the decision task of forming an accurate provisional diagnosis. GP(1) used five of nine modes of practice (intuitive/reflective/patient and peer-aided/system-aided e.g. ECG, and critical review of experiential and research evidence) described by Standing (2008). Critical review of experiential and research evidence involved assessing ecological and scientific validity (Chapter 5, Table 5.1) to review signs/symptoms true indication of an underlying illness, test hypotheses to exclude other conditions, and estimate the probability of pulmonary embolism.

Correspondence and coherence competence (Table 10.2) reflect perceptions of clinical decision-making (collaborative, experience/intuition, confidence, systematic, prioritizing, observation, standardized, reflective, ethical sensitivity, accountability) and conceptions of nursing (caring, listening/being there, practical procedures, knowledge/understanding, communicating, patience, teamwork, paperwork, empathizing and non-judgemental, professional) in the matrix model (Standing 2007a). This suggests that the process of clinical judgement/decision-making is very similar for doctors, nurses, and/or allied health professionals. Similarly, principles of nursing, such as caring, also appear applicable to medical and/or allied health professionals. Perhaps this is not surprising as integrated interprofessional healthcare and role flexibility are considered essential to achieve effective, patient-centred, coordinated whole systems working (Chapter 3). Doctors continue to have a key responsibility in diagnosing and treating patients with medical conditions and/or referring them to other practitioners, and GP(1) demonstrated excellence in this respect.

In theory it should have been easier for GP(2) to diagnose pulmonary embolism in 2007 than it was for GP(1) as I now had a history of the illness, symptoms were the same as before and, like before, their onset followed long-haul air travel, a known risk factor associated with pulmonary embolism. The fact that GP(2) incorrectly formed a provisional diagnosis of a chest infection highlights the uncertainty and difficulty of accurate decision-making, the health risks associated with mistakes, and the need to continually develop or enhance correspondence and coherence competence. GP(2) carried out a similar consultation and examination as described in Table 10.2 but on this occasion the pulse oximeter result was close to normal which could be the reason why pulmonary embolism was excluded. In 1997 I had driven to the surgery from work and the exertion exposed my reduced capacity to maintain normal blood oxygen saturation but in 2007 I was escorted to the surgery from home (did not exert myself) which may explain the different oximeter results. In truth neither GP had the equipment needed to confirm or refute pulmonary embolism so their provisional diagnoses served to determine whether they judged further specialist investigation was merited.

Tolerating false positive or false negative errors

There is, therefore, always an element of uncertainty in diagnostic decisions so errors are likely to occur. This means practitioners need to take account of potential consequences in the event their decisions might be wrong in order to minimize risks to patients in the resulting actions. Hammond (1996) referred to an inevitable duality of error which means that decision-makers have to choose between tolerating false negative or false positive errors and this needs to be reflected upon and considered in their decisions. For example, neither GP(1) nor GP(2) could be sure if I had a pulmonary embolism or not. GP(1) chose to tolerate false positive error (overestimating likelihood of pulmonary embolism) in the provisional diagnosis, not really knowing I had the illness. GP(2) chose to tolerate false negative error (underestimating likelihood of pulmonary embolism) in the provisional diagnosis, not really knowing I did not have the illness. Favouring false positive errors is a safer option but can result in hospitals being referred too many patients who do not need to be there which is not cost effective and may delay access to services by those who really need them. Favouring false negative errors carries more risks but avoids the problems of false positive errors.

GP(1)'s decision resulted in my immediate transfer by ambulance to hospital and if he had been proved wrong I would have been sent home after being assessed. GP(2)'s decision resulted in no immediate treatment as I was told to come back after 48 hours if I still felt unwell. This was a higher risk option in view of research evidence indicating pulmonary embolism is associated with significant mortality rates that are increased, as follows:

- If patient had pulmonary embolism before
- With every additional ten years of age
- If it is not treated immediately (Stein et al. 2004).

All of these risk factors applied to me and the following day I was taken to hospital after collapsing at work having climbed some stairs. My pulse oximeter blood oxygen saturation level was 70% which is below the critical level (75%) associated with maintaining healthy functioning of essential organs (Pagana and Pagana 2008). The false negative error made by GP(2) reflected lower levels of correspondence and coherence competence than demonstrated by GP(1) as the outcome was potentially life-threatening and the decision-making process lacked understanding of risk factors. This is also an example of the error of base rate neglect in being unaware of the relevant morbidity and mortality rates and/or a lack of critical analysis in applying them (Kahneman et al. 1982).

Case studies 1 and 2 indicate the variability of treatment patients can receive according to the different levels of expertise of healthcare practitioners attending to them. GP(1) was experienced while GP(2) was inexperienced which emphasizes the importance of informal work-based learning (Chapter 4) to build a repertoire of previous cases to learn from and apply skills as appropriate in future cases. GP(1) also demonstrated greater knowledge and understanding of relevant theory and research enabling a more considered and accurate risk assessment. This emphasizes the importance of formal learning in continuing professional development to update knowledge/skills. Informal learning helps develop practitioners' correspondence competence and formal learning helps develop practitioners' coherence competence. As illustrated in Table 10.2 safe and effective clinical judgement/decision-making requires using both contrasting and complementary skills sets. The educational and managerial implications of this are to create a common culture that promotes and integrates patient-centred care and practice-centred learning by every health professional. A reflexive-pragmatism model (Figure 10.1) is developed and presented later to meet this need.

Patient-centred versus task-oriented care

Advocating a philosophy of patient-centred care does not mean it is implemented in practice. For example, in Case study 1 (1997), on the third day I wanted to go to the bathroom and was told to stay in bed as this was normal procedure but the nurses (who were generally caring and attentive) could not explain why. This was an example of task-orientated rather than patient-centred care that did not correspond to my perceived needs, and also lacked coherence competence as no logical rationale was given for it. This triggered my interest in researching clinical decision-making and exploring how nurses learn to judge when standard procedures are applicable or when a new individualized variation is needed. Sometimes nurses deviated from procedures which they should adhere to because of mistaken prioritizing, for example, a nurse knew she should have washed hands and changed her disposable apron after a patient procedure but did not in case she was late serving lunch. This is an example of applying illogical or inappropriate decision rules (Cioffi and Markham 1997; Thompson 2002). In reflecting on my experience as a patient I concluded that:

- Task-orientated rather than patient-centred care was prevalent.
- Task-orientated care is not responsive to individual variations in patients' needs.
- Task-orientated care limits correspondence/coherence competence in decision-making.
- Task-orientated care constrains potential informal work-based learning opportunities.
- Task-orientated care is used to manage staff deployment in areas of high clinical demand.
- Task-orientated care delivers a low to moderate rather than a high quality service.

This experience reinforced the importance of transforming the clinical environment to promote a culture of both patient-centred care and practice-centred learning in interprofessional healthcare.

In Case study 2 (2007) nursing care remained task-orientated with limited correspondence or coherence competence evident and also lacked the caring aspect that I sensed before. This was unexpected as it occurred in the aftermath of NHS reform and reorganization intended to improve the quality and accountability of patient-centred, evidence-based care (Chapters 1–3). For example, in the emergency centre a doctor noticed my oxygen saturation level was too low and prescribed oxygen via a mask. I found the mask hard to tolerate for very long and kept removing it, and after a while the nurses stopped replacing it. When the doctor returned she expressed concern to two nurses sitting nearby that I was not getting sufficient oxygen, and one replied 'What can we do?' Naturally it was unwise of me to remove the oxygen mask but if you have breathing difficulties and low oxygen saturation you can, paradoxically, feel suffocated by the mask or become irritable and confused due to insufficient oxygenation of the brain. The nurses appeared to lack understanding of this, did not consider alternative ways of administering the oxygen, and implied it was my fault for not cooperating with the prescribed treatment.

After initial assessment at the emergency centre I spent four days in a 'clinical decision unit' which aims to provide further observation and assessment for up to 24 hours before transfer elsewhere. The fact that I was a patient there longer than usual may have detracted from the quality of care received as the nurses did not seem to include forming caring relationships or addressing patients' physical, psychological or social needs in the perception or performance their role. For example:

- My bed was allocated one pillow despite the fact that patients with respiratory problems require more pillows to elevate the chest and enhance breathing. I discovered a shortage occurred when patients were transferred because pillows went with them and were not replaced.
- When I experienced severe chest pain I pressed the buzzer, as instructed, to alert the nurses and request a painkiller, but it often took 20 minutes or more before someone responded.
- A male staff nurse approached me and, without addressing me or introducing himself or explaining his intentions, asked me to lie on my bed. When I asked why he said he had to give a prescribed injection. When I asked what it was, he could not tell me its name or its purpose.
- I was nauseous and vomited three times but no interest was shown in why it occurred, how it could be prevented, its effects on my dietary needs, and no fluid intake or output was recorded.
- I needed to go to the bathroom but it was busy so I asked a nurse if there was another one I could use who replied 'I don't know, I've only been here three days.'
- On the third day I approached the night sister and asked about a transfer to a medical ward. She simply ignored me, turned around, walked away and started talking to another nurse.

Unlike GP(1) in Table 10.2, the above examples demonstrate an absence of patient-centred care, correspondence or coherence competence, modes of practice in the revised cognitive continuum, or perceptions of clinical decision-making and conceptions of nursing identified in the matrix model. Perhaps this is because GP(1) has greater autonomy and control in clinical practice, patients are seen relatively briefly, and the work environment is more conducive to effective decision-making. In contrast, Case study 2 emergency centre and clinical decision unit nurses seemed unable to cope with the scale and intensity of clinical demands and this was exacerbated by the available skill-mix, staff numbers and use of inefficient procedures and practices. It appeared the nurses felt stressed and had little energy left for patients in their care so subconsciously dissociated from the responsibility. It echoed a study in the functioning of social systems as a defence against anxiety where staff depersonalize and dehumanize relations with patients to protect themselves from stress (Menzies 1960).

During the five days I was in hospital I lost half a stone in weight (from 8 to 7.5) and contracted a chest infection which exacerbated breathing difficulties associated with the pulmonary embolism, and delayed my recovery. The GP needed to prescribe three consecutive courses of different antibiotics to cure the persistent and resilient chest infection. I was grateful to the hospital doctors for their effective treatment and stabilization of my illness and felt the complications arose because of a delay in receiving treatment (due to incorrect provisional diagnosis from GP(2)) and the low standard of nursing care in the emergency centre and clinical decision unit. I asked one of the experienced GPs to inform GP(2) that I had a pulmonary embolism, not a chest infection (at that time), so he might learn from the experience and enhance his diagnostic skills. I also felt I had a responsibility to talk to the Director of Nursing about the quality of nursing, hoping something would be done to improve care for the benefit of other patients. It was agreed that I would present my 'lived experience' as a patient during a staff development event including those involved with and responsible for my care. The concerns I shared related to: communication and interpersonal skills, pain management, infection control, knowledge of drugs, caring for a patient suffering from a pulmonary embolism, positioning of patients with respiratory problems, dietary and fluid balance needs, relieving nausea/vomiting/constipation, and managing resources (including pillows). In effect this enacted the clinical audit/action research mode of practice (Standing 2008) to enhance patient-centred care by listening and learning from a patient's experience (Binnie and Titchen 1999).

Reflexive-pragmatism: complementary opposites in a lifelong learning cycle of patient-centred clinical judgement/ decision-making/interprofessional healthcare

Analysis of Case studies 1 and 2 demonstrates the importance of continuously applying a patient-centred philosophy in interprofessional clinical judgement/decision-making and that this requires lifelong practice-centred learning to maintain, amidst ongoing changes in healthcare. Successfully combining these processes enables integration of theory and practice resulting in the development and application of correspondence (practical) and coherence (logical) competence, exemplified by the clinical judgement/ decision-making of GP(1) in Table 10.2. Where this is not the case, a theory–practice gap (Maben et al. 2006) occurs, resulting in reduced levels of correspondence and coherence competence, less effective decision-making, and lower quality care. It is, therefore, incumbent upon policymakers, managers, practitioners and educators to create and maintain a culture combining patient-centred interprofessional healthcare and practice-centred learning. The reflexive-pragmatism model (Figure 10.1) is designed to represent and facilitate this process.

Figure 10.1 combines the theoretical perspectives in Chapters 1–5 within a single, unified, reflexive-pragmatism model where patient-centred care and lifelong practice-centred learning provide core values to continually energize, structure, and evaluate interprofessional healthcare. Doubled-headed arrows represent energizing (outward pointing) and grounding (inward pointing) clinical judgement/decision-making in the values of lifelong patient/ practice-centred care/learning. Pragmatism refers to lifelong learning in providing the highest possible standard of patient-centred care applying the best available evidence, techniques and resources to address problems in a specific context and timeframe. Reflexivity refers to lifelong learning in the critical self-examination of ideas, assumptions, biases and lack of knowledge or understanding that impede sound patient-centred clinical judgement/decision-making, and a commitment to improve knowledge and skills. Reflexive-pragmatism implies that these contrasting but complementary outward- and

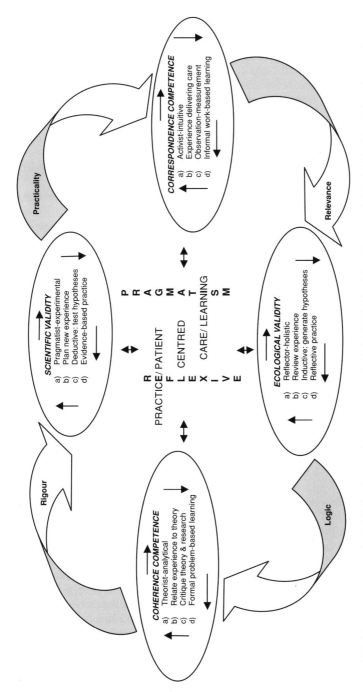

KEY: Coherence competence = Logical thinking; Correspondence competence = Practical skill; Scientific validity = Rigorous method; Ecological validity = Relevant interpretation

a) = Individual learning styles   b) = Experiential learning cycle   c) = Scientific research process   d) = Lifelong learning in and practising interprofessional healthcare

Figure 10.1 Reflexive-pragmatism: Logic, practicality, rigour and relevance in patient-centred, interprofessional clinical judgement and decision-making (Standing and Standing 2010)

215

inward-looking processes need to work together in a dynamic cycle of lifelong practice-centred learning, responsive to the constantly changing challenges of patient-centred interprofessional healthcare.

The four ovals in Figure 10.1 identify contrasting sets of practical or logical clinical judgement/decision-making skills (correspondence and coherence competence) and ways to assess relevance or rigour of experiential and theoretical knowledge (ecological and scientific validity). Examples of the application of these processes can be extracted from Table 10.2, as follows:

- GP(1) applied ecological validity to match patient account of illness with observation of patient (**relevance**).
- GP(1) applied scientific validity in testing hypotheses about possible causes of chest pain (**rigour**).
- GP(1) applied coherence competence to explain reason for referral in letter to duty doctor (**logic**).
- GP(1) applied correspondence competence to arrange urgent ambulance transfer to hospital (**practicality**).

Competence and validity are matched to different stages of four inter-related processes creating four dynamic subsystems (arrows denoting activity inside ovals, Figure 10.1) each of which is informed by and uniquely contributes to patient-centred care and practice-centred learning. The four processes that support each type of competence and validity in Figure 10.1 are as follows:

a)   Individual learning styles (Honey and Mumford 1998)
b)   Experiential learning cycle (Kolb 1984)
c)   Scientific research process (Wallace 1978)
d)   Learning/practising healthcare (Standing 2007b).

Honey and Mumford (1998) linked four individual learning styles (a) to corresponding stages of Kolb's (1984) experiential learning cycle (b). This helped to highlight learning preferences and strengths, educational benefits of interactive teaching methods, how an experiential cycle enables application of alternative learning styles, and how it complemented the notion of practitioners being 'knowledgeable-doers' (Benner 1984). However, this is limited in developing analytic decision-making skills so corresponding stages of Wallace's (1978) scientific research process (c) were added and linked to learning/practising evidence-based and reflective, patient centred decision-making (d) in a reflective-pragmatism model (Standing 2007b). The reflexive-pragmatism model, developed here (Figure 10.1), adds key concepts from cognitive continuum theory to integrate a), b), c) and d) and provide a more effective tool to guide, develop, apply and evaluate decision-making. Reflexivity is linked with maintaining rigour, controlling researcher bias (Dowling 2006) and high levels of critical self-evaluation. Coherence and correspondence competence (Hammond 1996, Standing 2008), scientific (Kahneman et al. 1982) and ecological validity (Brunswik 1956) represent defining and contrasting decision-making processes used to collate (a), (b), (c) and (d) in their respective subsystems. These are interconnected (large arrows) in a continuous cycle of interprofessional patient-centred clinical decision-making and practice-centred learning.

An emphasis on reflexivity and practice-centred learning reinforces the place of individual learning styles in the reflexive-pragmatism model since correspondence/coherence competence and ecological/scientific validity in clinical judgement/decision-making involve developing and applying each style, as appropriate. Table 10.3 relates the individual learning styles to associated strengths and potential weaknesses in clinical decision-making.

Table 10.3 Relating individual learning styles to clinical decision-making

Learning style	Associated strengths	Potential weaknesses
Activist-intuitive	Learning by getting on with what needs to be done Able to cope with unpredictable events	Making rash decisions
Reflector-holistic	Reflective learning from previous experience Able to use imagination to visualize new possibilities	Slow at making decisions
Theorist-analytical	Learning through academic study or reading literature Able to grasp relevant theoretical perspectives	Over-complicating decisions
Pragmatist-experimental	Learning by testing out ideas in practice Able to identify priorities and makes plans to achieve them	Over-simplifying decisions

---

Reflective activity 10.2

1. Refer to Table 10.3, reflect on the descriptions of individual learning styles, and identify which one (or combination) most closely represents your style. Write down the reason why you think this is the case and give an example.
2. Ask some of your colleagues to do the same exercise independently. At this point everyone has their own self-assessment that they have not shared with others.
3. Then each person peer-assesses what they think the preferred learning style is of each other member in your group of colleagues, stating why and using examples.
4. Exchange peer-assessments, compare with self-assessments, note similarities and/or differences and review each other's reasons and/or evidence for choices made.

5. Discuss the associated strengths and potential weaknesses of the different styles in relation to clinical decision-making, and reflect on how these may apply to you.
6. Each person then chooses a style they would like to develop further and identifies an activity to practise using it. Agree a time to meet again to review progress. If you are stuck for ideas, ask advice from someone adept in the style you want to practise.

In the historical development of healthcare education key qualities associated with decision-making have been enabled at different times, such as learning procedures (practicality), theory (logic), reflective practice (relevance), and evidence-based practice (rigour). Reflexive-pragmatism offers a vision to co-ordinate the application of these qualities. Imagine a rally car negotiating the slippery, uneven, unpredictable terrain of health and illness with an engine of patient-centred care that drives all four wheels (correspondence competence, coherence competence, ecological validity, and scientific validity) simultaneously. Engaging one or two wheels will not provide enough grip and the quality of clinical judgement/decision-making in nursing and inter-professional healthcare will reflect this. Sustainable refuelling via practice-centred learning maintains momentum. Case studies 1 and 2 gave examples of high and low quality care showing how it can be done well and what can be improved. Reflexive-pragmatism applies progressive education values of empowerment via lifelong learning in applying problem solving skills for personal development and social functioning (Dewey 1938) that was influenced by William James's (1842–1910) philosophy of pragmatism. Table 10.4 offers practitioners a checklist to self assess correspondence and coherence competence ecological and scientific validity, and patient-centred values in a reflexive-pragmatism model for 2010.

Summary

This chapter has included an autobiographical account of receiving acute medical care which provided the basis to evaluate practitioners' clinical decision-making, and the ways that such skills can be enhanced. Examples of good practice in applying correspondence competence used practical and interpersonal skills to listen, observe, elicit information, physically examine and inform diagnostic and treatment decisions relevant to patient needs, and achieve good outcomes of care. There was also evidence of cross-referencing information cues such as relating pallor, breathing difficulty, and chest pain exacerbated by moderate exertion, and checking the ecological validity or relevance of interpretations regarding symptoms. Examples of good practice in applying coherence competence used logical thinking to guide system-atic problem solving, understand implications of observations in relation to theory and research, assess risks, and prioritize clinical decisions. There was also evidence of checking scientific validity or rigour in testing and

Table 10.4 Reflexive-pragmatism: logic, practicality, rigour and relevance – a checklist

	Reflexive	*Pragmatism*
Summary	Critical self-examination of thinking processes, biases and limitations in knowledge that impair judgement, and ongoing commitment to improve skills	Critical awareness applied in continually assessing changes in practice settings, recognizing implications for patient care, and taking action to address problems
Skills	*Coherence competence* Logical decision-making skills: sound knowledge of relevant theory and research enabling understanding of health, illness, treatment principles; applying systematic problem solving, recognize significance of risk factors; ability to explain, justify and defend decisions verbally and in writing	*Correspondence competence* Practical decision-making skills: accurate observation, and perception via senses, communicating, listening; eliciting information to ensure decisions are relevant to patient's needs during assessment and treatment; carry out skilled procedures to achieve high quality care outcomes for the patient
Tests of rigour and relevance	*Scientific validity* What theoretical or evidence base supports your decision? How did you test application of theory or research? Why did you reject other options?	*Ecological validity* How do you know your observations truly reflect the patient's health status? What different indicators can you use to assess patient's response to treatment?
Professional values and ethical code e.g. NMC (2008) NB non-nurses/ midwives can substitute here extracts of own professional ethical code	'As a professional, you are personally accountable for actions and omissions in your practice and must always be able to justify your decisions' (p. 1) 'You must deliver care based on the best available evidence or best practice' (p. 7) 'You must keep your knowledge and skills up to date throughout your working life' (p. 7)	'You must listen to the people in your care and respond to their concerns and preferences' (p. 3) 'You must be able to demonstrate that you have acted in someone's best interest if you have provided care in an emergency' (p. 4) 'You must confirm that the outcome of any delegated task meets required standards' (p. 6)

discounting hypotheses regarding alternative possible causes of symptoms, such as an ECG to assess heart function. Conversely, errors were related to lower levels of the above skills due to less knowledgeable or experienced practitioners, and organizational or staffing issues in areas of high clinical demand, and what Maben et al. (2006) referred to as a theory–practice gap in clinical practice.

As outlined above, effective clinical judgement/decision-making involves using both practical and logical skills, and assessing the rigour and relevance of available evidence. This process is dependent on integrating theory and practice which the examples of good practice demonstrated. In reflecting on ways to enhance the integration of theory–practice in clinical decision-making, a new reflexive-pragmatism model was developed, incorporating the above concepts, and relating them to both patient-centred care and life-long practice-centred learning in interprofessional healthcare. It is hoped that such a model offers a shared philosophy of both healthcare practice and interprofessional education that represents a step towards bridging a theory–practice gap referred to by Maben et al. (2006). Reflective activities encouraged practitioners' critical self-assessment (reflexivity) of professional development needs in clinical judgement/decision-making, and a 'reflexive-pragmatism' checklist was provided, summarizing key skills, processes and values, and how to assess them.

Key points

- Understanding patients' experience/perspective of their illness/healthcare received is vital to assess the *relevance* of assessment information/treatment plans within patient-centred care.
- *Practical* skills (observing patients, communicating, listening, checking vital signs, using aids e.g. ECG, clinical procedures) are needed for accurate assessment/evaluating care outcomes.
- *Logical* skills (applying theory and research in a systematic way to recognize significance of observations and healthcare implications) are needed to explain, justify and defend decisions.
- Planning/delivering high quality care, relevant to patients' needs, applying logical principles, requires *rigour* to test hypotheses e.g. causes of chest pain, and evidence base for decisions.
- Technical terms for above knowledge/skills are: *ecological* validity (relevance), *correspondence* competence (practicality), *coherence* competence (logic) and *scientific* validity (rigour).
- Accurate/safe/effective clinical judgement/decision-making is a complex process that combines and applies high levels of correspondence/coherence competence and ecological/scientific validity.
- Uncertainty is never totally eliminated so errors occur in underestimating risks (false negative) or overestimating risks (false positive) and decision-makers need to plan contingencies for this.

- Task-orientated-basic care, is provided in areas of high clinical demand which discourages use of critical thinking, correspondence/coherence competence and ecological/scientific validity.
- High workload, inadequate staff numbers/skill mix and inefficient procedures/use of resources lead to a stressed workforce lacking in decision-making competence or caring qualities.
- *Reflexive-pragmatism* = patient/practice-centred model of interprofessional healthcare/lifelong learning that combines correspondence/coherence competence and ecological/scientific validity.

References

Benner, P. (1984) *From Novice to Expert*. Menlo Park, CA: Addison-Wesley.

Binnie, A. and Titchen, A. (1999) *Freedom to Practise: The development of patient-centred nursing*. Oxford: Butterworth-Heinemann.

Brunswik, E. (1956) *Perception and the Representative Design of Psychological Experiments*, 2nd edn. Berkeley: University of California Press.

Cioffi, J. and Markham, R. (1997) Clinical decision-making: managing complexity. *Journal of Advanced Nursing*, 25: 265–72.

Dewey, J. (1938) *Experience and Education*. London: Collier Macmillan.

Dowling, M. (2006) Approaches to reflexivity in qualitative research. *Nurse Researcher*, 13(3): 7–21.

Hammond, K.R. (1996) *Human Judgment and Social Policy: Irreducible uncertainty, inevitable error, unavoidable injustice*. New York: Oxford University Press.

Honey, P. and Mumford, A. (1998) Setting the scene for learning styles, in C.M. Downie and P. Basford (eds) *Teaching and Assessing in Clinical Practice*. London: University of Greenwich.

Kahneman, D., Slovic, P. and Tversky, A. (eds) (1982) *Judgment under Uncertainty: Heuristics and biases*. Cambridge: Cambridge University Press.

Kolb, D.A. (1984) *Experiential Learning*. Englewood Cliffs, NJ: Prentice-Hall.

Maben, J., Latter, S. and Macleod Clark, J, (2006) The theory-practice gap: impact of professional-bureaucratic work conflict on newly-qualified nurses. *Journal of Advanced Nursing*, 55(4): 465–77.

Menzies, I. (1960) *The Structuring of Social Systems as a Defence against Anxiety*. London: Tavistock Institute.

Nursing and Midwifery Council (NMC) (2008) *The Code: Standards for conduct, performance and ethics for nurses and midwives*. London: NMC.

Pagana, K. and Pagana, T. (2008) *Mosby's Diagnostic and Laboratory Test Reference*, 9th edn. St Louis: Mosby.

Standing, M. (2007a) Clinical decision-making skills on the developmental journey from student to Registered Nurse: a longitudinal inquiry. *Journal of Advanced Nursing*, 60(3): 257–69.

Standing, M. (2007b) Reflective-pragmatism: complementary opposites in a dynamic cycle of learning – A curriculum model to enhance integrated theory-practice. Core Paper, *Nurse Education Tomorrow*, 18th Annual International Conference, University of Cambridge.

Standing, M. (2008) Clinical judgement and decision-making in nursing – nine modes of practice in a revised cognitive continuum. *Journal of Advanced Nursing*, 62(1): 124–34.

Stein, P.D., Kayali, F. and Olson, R.E. (2004) Regional differences in rates of diagnosis and mortality of pulmonary thromboembolism. *American Journal of Cardiology,* 93: 1194–97.

Thompson, C. (2002) Human error, bias, decision making and judgement in nursing: the need for a systematic approach, in C. Thompson and D. Dowding (eds) *Clinical Decision Making and Judgement in Nursing.* Edinburgh: Churchill Livingstone.

Wallace, W. (1978) An overview of elements in the scientific process, in J. Bynner and K. Stribley (eds) *Social Research: Principles and procedures.* Harlow: Longman with Oxford University Press.

Conclusion

It is now time to review the contents of *Clinical Judgement and Decision-making: Nursing and Interprofessional Healthcare*, summarize the themes discussed, and draw conclusions about the book. A What? So what? Now what? (Driscoll 2000) format is used to structure the conclusion.

What?

Chapters 1–5 discussed: i) research-based matrix model of nurses' perceptions of decision-making; ii) literature review of advanced practitioners' qualities and role; iii) applying whole systems theory in patient-centred/integrated healthcare; iv) informal/formal lifelong learning for healthcare practitioners; and v) cognitive continuum theory relating variations in decision tasks to different modes of practice. Chapters 6–10 applied aspects of theories to analyse practitioners' clinical judgement/decision-making in real case studies, and a reflexive-pragmatism model was created by combining various contrasting and complementary theoretical perspectives.

Complementary opposites

Tacit knowledge – embodied, embedded	Explicit knowledge – theory, research
Informal learning – incidental, work-based	Formal learning – structured, university-based
Professional knowing-in-action/ practice	Deliberation, technical/calculative rationality
Creative thinking – inductive process	Critical thinking – deductive process
Descriptive/observational decision theory	Normative/statistical, prescriptive theory
Intuitive/experiential decision-making	Analytic/rational decision-making
Experiential and reflective cycle	Systematic problem solving cycle
Reflective practice – local focus	Evidence-based practice – national focus
Correspondence competence – practical	Coherence competence – logical
Ecological validity – testing relevance	Scientific validity – testing rigour
Pragmatism – optimize care outcome	Reflexivity – self-review of biases

The reflexive-pragmatism model (Chapter 10, Figure 10.1) was created to unify complementary opposites identified above into a coherent 'whole system' of clinical judgement/decision-making in patient-centred, interprofessional healthcare and lifelong practice-centred learning.

So what?

There are limitations to what any book can achieve if it does not give readers a strong enough incentive to pick it up in the first place or gives too great an incentive not to pick it up again! In the introduction it claimed to enable readers to access current and relevant theory and demonstrate how it could be applied to practice. In considering whether readers feel this promise has/has not been kept, reference is made to their potential individual learning styles (Honey and Mumford 1998).

Individual learning styles – book appeal

Theorist-analytical

A range of theory and research was critically discussed including Bayes' theorem, advanced practice, complex whole systems, and learning processes. Cognitive continuum theory showed how opposing theories can be combined to compensate for each other's limitations. The creation of a new reflexive-pragmatism model may also interest such readers.

Pragmatist-experimental

A variety of practitioners' accounts of their clinical practice were used to show how the different perspectives could be applied. It may be helpful to emulate this process if required to apply theory to practice for assessments during continuing professional development programmes. The activities also give such readers opportunities to test the usefulness of concepts.

Activist-intuitive

The structure of the book enables scanning via overviews, objectives, key points and summaries so that some useful information can be gleaned relatively quickly. A number of diagrams summarize important information visually, providing a relief from constant text. The book also encourages lecturers to engage such readers in participative learning and teaching methods.

Reflector-holistic

Learning by reflecting upon experience was endorsed throughout the book: the matrix model was the product of nurses' reflections; the Lens model showed how to analyse and validate observations in practice; cognitive continuum theory was adapted to include reflective judgement; and the book encourages mentoring and clinical supervision to support practitioners.

The book appears, therefore, to have included material relevant to its aims, and the needs of a broad cross-section of readers. Regrettably, it was not feasible to include every clinical area in the book but it is hoped that such practitioners find they are able to apply the decision-making content.

Now what?

Books take a long time to produce and so it is important to assess this book's currency and relevance regarding anticipated developments in healthcare. National Health Service (NHS) reform is expected to continue in order to achieve the goal of an accessible, safe, effective, integrated, locally accountable, high quality patient-centred service (Darzi 2007). This book has discussed, developed and applied tools to guide and evaluate safe, accurate, effective clinical judgement and decision-making which are responsive and relevant to patients' needs. It is, therefore, topical and may be used as an instrument contributing to the achievement of the above goals. Similarly, education developments mirror NHS reform in equipping nurses and other health professionals with the knowledge and skills associated with providing the service envisaged. For example, increase required academic level for entry as a registered nurse from diploma to degree, prepare practitioners for more specialist roles, and prioritize interprofessional education (Longley et al. 2007). This book acknowledges a symbiosis between theory and practice, recognizing the importance of optimizing informal work-based/formal university-based education through lifelong learning. Indeed, the new reflexive-pragmatism model makes explicit links between rigorous and relevant patient-centred care and practice-centred learning in clinical judgement and decision-making and interprofessional healthcare, as follows (extract from Chapter 10, p. 214):

> Pragmatism refers to lifelong learning in providing the highest possible standard of patient-centred care, applying the best available evidence, techniques and resources to address problems in a specific context and timeframe. Reflexivity refers to lifelong learning in the critical self-examination of ideas, assumptions, biases, and lack of knowledge or understanding that impede sound patient-centred clinical judgement/decision-making, and, a commitment to improve knowledge and skills.

The reflexive-pragmatism model is, recommended for use by and consistency between policy-makers, managers, educators and practitioners in creating and sustaining a shared culture that is conducive to effective clinical judgement and decision-making in nursing and interprofessional healthcare.

References

Darzi, A. (2007) *Our NHS, Our Future.* Interim Report. London: Department of Health.

Driscoll, J. (2000) *Practising Clinical Supervision: A reflective approach.* Edinburgh: Bailliere Tindall.

Honey, P. and Mumford, A. (1998) Setting the scene for learning styles, in C.M. Downie and P. Basford (eds) *Teaching and Assessing in Clinical Practice.* London: University of Greenwich.

Longley, M. et al. (2007) *Nursing: Towards 2015.* London: Nursing and Midwifery Council.

Glossary

Activity theory When individuals interact with others or the environment, they create tools (cultural artefacts) such as documents, representing mental processes which become accessible to others.

Advanced practitioner Experienced clinical professional with advanced knowledge and skills empowered to make high-level clinical decisions, manage caseloads and/or areas of practice.

Analytic/rational decision theory Human judgement is unreliable due to inherent bias. Research experiments are the best way to minimize bias (identify independent and dependent variables; hypothesize/test cause/effect relationship in controlled laboratory setting) where the results are analysed using statistical probabilities and tests of their predictive value and margins of error.

Clinical decision-making Complex process of observation, information processing, critical thinking, evaluating evidence, applying knowledge, problem solving, reflection, judgement to select best option from available choices to optimize patients' health and minimize potential harm.

Clinical judgement Applying different sources of information derived from observing or listening to patients, feedback from others, measurements and investigations, and drawing conclusions.

Cognitive continuum theory Practice-based integrated decision theory where a system of low to highly structured decision tasks prompts a system of cognition ranging from intuition to analysis to select a mode of response that best matches the demands of the current problem.

Coherence competence Logical, systematic, consistent, open to scrutiny, retraceable process.

Community of practice People with common goals interacting in groups and striving to achieve them.

Complex adaptive systems Diverse, independent, potentially entangled or chaotic entities that are capable of 'untangling' in an interdependent collaborative response to perceived new challenges.

Correspondence competence   Practical, accurate observation, skilful action and effective outcome.

Creative thinking   Observation, analysis, storing concepts, searching for associations, and generating new ideas using different techniques (analogies, random word association, classic 'brainstorming').

Critical thinking   Purposeful, self-regulatory judgement using interpretation, analysis, evaluation, drawing conclusions and explaining supporting evidence.

Descriptive models   Observing, describing and analysing (for example, using 'thinking aloud' technique) how decisions are made by practitioners and/or managers in their professional roles.

Ecological validity   Identified information cues truly represent hidden characteristics that inferences relate to.

Embedded knowledge   Contextual and cultural collaborative understanding of social and/or political systems, local customs, values, and their shared routines or working practices.

Embodied knowledge   Personal understanding, sensory, psychomotor (practical), affective (emotional) and interpersonal skills associated with experience and intuition.

Embrained knowledge   Capacity to process and evaluate information using systematic problem solving, reflection, and critical and creative thinking skills.

Encoded knowledge   Theory, research, applied physical and social sciences, professional and ethical code, health/social care policy, standardized procedures, clinical guidelines and legislation.

Expansive learning   Complex form of lifelong learning that does not separate individual from organizational learning, and that focuses on continuous transformation to face new challenges.

Experiential learning cycle   Experience, reflect/review, relate to theory, plan ahead, repeat cycle.

Explicit knowledge   Conscious encoded/articulated content and analytic/embrained process.

Force field analysis   Planning transformation from present to future state involving mapping/assessing contradictory forces blocking energy and make changes so that positive forces outweigh negative ones.

Individual preferred learning styles   Theorist/analytical (academic study), pragmatist/experimental (testing out possibilities), activist/intuitive (committing to action), reflector/holistic (reviewing experience).

Intuitive/experiential decision theory   Judgement is a product of interaction between individual and environment and cannot be understood by studying either in isolation. Humans are goal-directed but surrounded by uncertainty and their perceptual accuracy is prone to error so they use range of information cues to make sense of social contexts and 'weigh up' best option in decision-making.

Knowing-in-action   Competent practitioners usually know more than they can say. Evidence of such tacit (embodied knowledge) is obtained by observing practitioners in their daily work.

Knowing-in-practice   Lifelong learning is 'situated' and needs to be understood in relation to the clinical context where it is generated and/or applied. It is socially constructed embodied/embedded professional knowledge that cannot be reduced to component parts or abstractly represented.

Legitimate peripheral participation   People need to be accepted in order to join a community of practice. New members are allowed to practise simple or low-risk tasks that are productive in some way. Participation means they gradually learn to take part in all aspects of community life.

Lens model   Reality perceived through an interpretive 'lens' where many observable information cues are 'weighted' and used to make inferences about assumed underlying characteristics.

Normative models   Rational, logical, scientific, evidence-based decisions informed by statistical analysis of experimental/survey research representative of population to which findings apply.

Pragmatism   Lifelong learning in providing the highest possible standard of patient-centred care, applying the best available evidence, techniques and resources, to address identified problems in a specific clinical context and timeframe.

Prescriptive models   Frameworks, guidelines, assessment tools or algorithms designed to enhance clinical decisions, for example, NICE guidelines.

Problem solving cycle   Notice discrepancy between current and desired situation, specify problem, identify goals, make realistic plans to achieve them, take required action, and review the results.

'PROFESSIONAL' taxonomy   Informal work-based learning: **P** Practice and repetition, **R** Reflection, **O** Observing and copying, **F** Feedback, **E** Extra-occupational transfer, **S** Stretching activities, **S** Switching perspectives, **I** Interaction with coach, **O** Osmosis, **N** Neurological/psychological devices/techniques, **A** Articulation, **L** Liaison/collaboration (Cheetham and Chivers 2001).

Reflexive-pragmatism   Model applying concepts from cognitive continuum theory (coherence/logic and correspondence/practical competence, and ecological/relevance and scientific/rigour validity) linking patient-centred care and lifelong practice-centred learning in clinical judgement/decision-making within interprofessional healthcare (see also reflexivity and pragmatism).

Reflexivity   Lifelong learning in the critical self-examination of ideas, assumptions, biases and any lack of knowledge or understanding that may impede sound patient-centred clinical judgement and decision-making, plus a commitment to take action and improve knowledge and skills.

Repertoires of solutions   Informal work-based participative learning ranging from simple to more complex activities that builds upon existing mental models, derived from previous experience.

Scientific research process   Critique existing theory and research, deduce hypotheses, test hypotheses, observe and measure results, generate new hypotheses as necessary, repeat cycle.

Scientific validity   Rigorous selection/control of variables, experiment to test cause/effect relations.

Supervision   Restorative/supportive (emotional support to cope with work related stress), formative/educational (reflection and development of knowledge and skills), normative/managerial (monitoring the effectiveness and quality of clinical practice) guidance from a trusted, experienced colleague.

Tacit knowledge   Subconscious/unconscious embodied/embedded content and intuitive/embrained process.

Technical rationality   Applying explicit encoded knowledge from reliable authorities or objective quantifiable information sources to explain events and/or develop practitioners', understanding.

Whole systems theory   Healthcare and social care practitioners collaborate to dispel traditional professional boundaries and integrate interprofessional, patient/user consultation in their practice.

Index

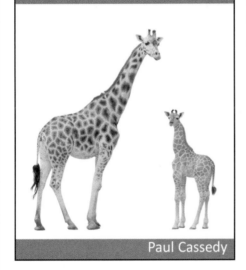

FIRST STEPS IN CLINICAL SUPERVISION

A Guide for Healthcare Professionals

Paul Cassedy

9780335236510 (Paperback)
November 2010

eBook also available

This practical book is designed as a toolkit for anyone starting out as a clinical supervisor. The book focuses on developing core skills of supervision, as well as your ability to reflect and improve on those skills.

Addressing all aspects of supervision, the book gives you practical frameworks needed to start, maintain and evaluate clinical supervision - from how to start a supervision contract to how to run a session.

Key features:

- Clear information and guidance on what the supervisor needs to know as they prepare to take on the role of clinical supervisor
- Practical examples and demonstration of key clinical supervision skills
- Simple explanations of the key frameworks and models for clinical supervision

www.openup.co.uk

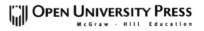 OPEN UNIVERSITY PRESS
McGraw · Hill Education

THE NURSE MENTOR AND REVIEWER UPDATE BOOK

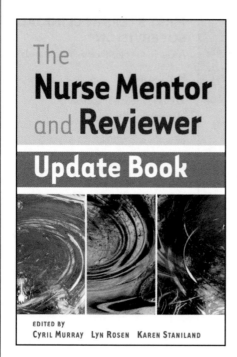

Cyril Murray, Lyn Rosen and
  Karen Staniland
9780335241194 (Paperback)
2010

eBook also available

This practical and flexible guide explains the meaning of competence and is designed to help mentors judge competence in line with Nursing and Midwifery Council standards and the NHS Knowledge and Skills Framework.

Key features:

- Designed to help mentors judge their own competence against national standards
- Supports qualified mentors in meeting the evidence required for annual updates
- A range of activities are included to help support the mentoring process to provide a range of different sources of evidence at appraisal interviews

www.openup.co.uk

OPEN UNIVERSITY PRESS
McGraw - Hill Education